FAT TO FIT WEIGHTLOSS MANUAL

Unbelievable Transformation: Lose 30 Pounds of Fat in 30 Days

Dr. Barnett Wright

Copyright © 2020 [Dr. Barnett Wright]

Without the publisher's authorization, no part of this publication may be copied, stored, or transmitted in any way, including by printing, recording, or other electronic or mechanical methods, except brief quotations used in critical reviews and other noncommercial uses allowed by copyright law.

No part of this book may be reproduced in any form or by any means, including photocopying, recording, or electronic methods, or be stored in a retrieval system or transmitted.

Table of Contents

Introduction

James was a thirty-year-old man who had struggled with his weight his entire life. He had tried every diet and exercise program out there and nothing seemed to work. He was desperate to find something that would finally help him shed the extra pounds.

One day he stumbled across a website with a manual on how to lose 30 pounds in 30 days. Even though he had his doubts, he chose to give it a shot. This manual outlined an intense diet and exercise plan that promised to help him reach his goal.

James was determined to make it work, so he followed the plan to the letter. He cut out all processed foods and fast food from his diet and instead focused on eating fresh and healthy fruits and vegetables. He also started exercising every day.

At first, the weight didn't seem to be coming off, but James kept pushing forward. After the first week, he noticed a difference. He had lost nearly 10 pounds. He kept going and by the end of the month, he had lost 30 pounds!

James was ecstatic. He had finally achieved his weight loss goal and was feeling better than ever. He was so proud of himself for sticking with the plan and achieving his goal.

James was so inspired by his success that he decided to keep going. He changed his diet and exercise routine to maintain his new weight and also started to share his story with others. Soon, he was inspiring many others to make a lifestyle change and achieve their own weight loss goals.

James was living proof that you can achieve anything you set your mind to. He had lost 30 pounds in 30 days and he was determined to never gain it back.

Chapter 1

Weight Loss and its Benefits

Weight loss is the process of reducing body weight by reducing fat and/or increasing muscle mass. It can be accomplished either by food or exercise, or both. Weight loss can have many benefits, including improved health, increased confidence, and a more attractive appearance.

Weight loss can improve health by reducing the risk of health conditions such as diabetes, heart disease, and high blood pressure. Weight loss can also improve energy levels, reduce stress, and improve sleep quality. Furthermore, weight loss can increase self-confidence and self-esteem.

When it comes to exercise, the type of activity should be tailored to individual fitness levels and goals. Aerobic exercises, such as walking, running, biking, swimming, and dancing, are great for burning calories and improving metabolism. Strength-training exercises, such as weight lifting and bodyweight exercises, can help to build muscle, burn fat, and improve overall health.

Finally, diet plays an important role in weight loss. Eating a well-balanced diet with plenty of fruits, vegetables, lean proteins, and healthy fats can help to provide the body with the nutrients it needs to stay healthy and support weight loss. Limiting portion sizes and avoiding processed foods can also help to reduce calorie intake and promote weight loss.

In summary, weight loss can have many benefits, including improved health, increased confidence, and a more attractive appearance. It can be achieved through diet and exercise, and it is important to tailor these to individual fitness levels and goals. Eating a balanced diet and limiting portion sizes can also help to promote weight loss.

Planning Your Weight Loss Diet

When you're planning your weight loss diet, it's important to consider your lifestyle and your goals. What kind of diet will work best for you? Do you have any health conditions that need to be taken into account?

The first step is to figure out how many calories you need to consume each day to reach your goal. This number should be determined by your age, gender, height, and activity level. It's important to track your caloric intake to stay on track with your diet goals.

Once you know how many calories you need to eat each day, it's time to plan your meals. Ensure that you are consuming the proper ratio of proteins, carbs, fats, and fibre. Make sure to include plenty of fresh fruits and vegetables in your diet, as well as healthy proteins such as fish and lean meats.

You should also consider adding physical activity to your weight loss diet. Exercise can help you reach your goals faster and can help you maintain a healthy weight. You may also want to consider adding supplements to your diet to help you reach your goals.

Finally, it's important to remember that a weight loss diet is not a "quick fix" and you should be prepared to make lifelong changes to reach and maintain your desired weight. Be sure to seek advice from a doctor or nutritionist if you're unsure about any aspect of your diet. With the proper planning and dedication, you can create a weight-loss loss diet that works for you

Creating a Healthy Eating Plan
Creating a healthy eating plan can be a daunting task, especially if you are new to the process. However, it is an Important step to take to maintain a healthy lifestyle some tips to help you get started:

1. Start by assessing your current eating habits. Take some time to reflect on what you are currently eating and consider any changes you would like to make.

2. Set realistic goals. Make sure that the goals you set are achievable and don't set yourself up for failure.

3. Make a plan. Think about what meals and snacks you will include in your eating plan and make a shopping list accordingly.

4. Focus on nutrient-rich foods. Aim to include plenty of fresh fruits and vegetables, lean protein, whole grains, and healthy fats in your diet.

5. Incorporate physical activity. Exercise is an important part of maintaining a healthy lifestyle and should be included in your plan.

6. Get support. Friends, family, or a nutrition expert can help you stay on track with your plan and provide encouragement.

By following these steps, you can create a healthy eating plan that is tailored to your individual needs. Remember, it is important to stay consistent and make small changes over time.

Increase Physical Activity

Increasing physical activity is a great way to improve your overall health and well-being. Regular physical activity can help you maintain a healthy weight, reduce your risk of chronic diseases, and improve your mood.

There are many ways to increase physical activity. Start by making small changes to your daily routine. Take the stairs instead of the elevator or escalator, or park further away from your destination. You can also take a walk during your lunch break, or take a dance class with friends.

You can also set a goal for yourself. Set a goal to walk or run a certain number of miles each week, or to do a certain number of push-ups or sit-ups each day. Once you reach your goal, reward yourself with something special.

If you're having trouble getting started, sign up for a class or join a gym. Having an instructor or trainer to motivate you can make it easier to stay on track.

Finally, don't forget to rest and refuel. Make sure to get enough sleep and eat nutritious meals to give your body the energy it needs for physical activity.

Increasing physical activity is an important part of leading a healthy lifestyle. By making small changes to your routine, setting goals, and taking breaks when needed, you can make physical activity a regular part of your life.

In conclusion

Increasing physical activity is an important part of leading a healthy lifestyle. It can help you maintain a healthy weight, reduce your risk of chronic diseases, and improve your mood. Start by making small changes to your everyday routine, and set goals to stay motivated. Sign up for a class or join a gym if you need help getting started. Finally, don't forget to rest and refuel with plenty of sleep and nutritious meals.

Establishing Realistic Goals
Weight loss and diet goals should be individualised and tailored to your specific needs and situation. To ensure success, it is important to set realistic goals that can be achieved in a reasonable amount of time. Here are some tips for setting realistic weight loss and diet goals:

1. Start with small changes. Don't attempt to adjust your diet drastically all at once. Start with small, achievable changes, such as swapping out sugary drinks for water or replacing unhealthy snacks with healthier options.

2. Set specific goals. Instead of setting a vague goal such as "I want to lose weight," make it more specific. Like I want to lose 10 pounds in one week.

3. Break your goals down into manageable chunks. Instead of setting one long-term goal, break it down into smaller goals that can be achieved in a shorter amount of time.

4. Choose achievable goals. Setting goals that are too ambitious can lead to frustration and disappointment if they are not achieved. Pick possible goals

5. Focus on nutrition. Instead of focusing on weight loss, focus on improving your overall nutrition. Eating more whole foods, such as fruits and vegetables, and cutting down on processed and sugary foods, can help you achieve a healthier lifestyle.

6. Track your progress. Monitoring your progress is an important part of achieving your goals. Track your dietary consumption and exercise using a food diary or an app.

7. Reward yourself. Achieving small goals is an excellent way to stay motivated and on track. Celebrate your successes by rewarding yourself with something special.

8. Get support. Surround yourself with a supportive network of family, friends, and healthcare professionals who can encourage and motivate you.

By setting realistic goals and using these tips, you can achieve your weight loss and diet goals.

Chapter 2

Understanding Macronutrients

The nutrients that provide the body energy are called macronutrients. These include protein, carbohydrates, and fat. When dieting for weight loss, macronutrients are important to consider to ensure that the body is getting the necessary nutrients for health and weight loss.

For weight loss, it is recommended to get the majority of your calories from lean sources of protein, complex carbohydrates, and healthy fats. Eating meals that contain the right macronutrients can help to keep you feeling full and satisfied, and can also help to keep blood sugar levels balanced.

Carbohydrates are the main source of energy for the body and are broken down into glucose, which is then used to fuel the body's metabolic processes. Carbohydrates are found in foods like grains, fruits, vegetables, and dairy products.

When consumed in moderation, carbohydrates can help to keep blood sugar levels stable, provide energy, and maintain a healthy weight.

Protein is an essential macronutrient for weight loss and dieting. It is important for building lean muscle mass, which helps to burn more calories and increase metabolism. Protein can be found in foods like lean meats, eggs, nuts, and legumes. Eating high-protein foods can help to increase satiety, which can lead to fewer calories consumed overall.

Fat is an important macronutrient for weight loss and dieting. It helps to slow down digestion and keep you feeling full for longer. Healthy fats, such as those found in avocados, olive oil, nuts, and fatty fish, can help to provide essential fatty acids and vitamins to the body. Eating healthy fats in moderation can help to promote weight loss and improve overall health.

Overall, understanding macronutrients are essential for successful weight loss and dieting. Eating a balanced diet that includes a variety of carbohydrates, proteins, and healthy fats can help to provide the body with the necessary nutrients and energy needed to sustain life and aid in weight loss.

Food Choices

When it comes to weight loss, food choices play a major role in achieving your desired results. Eating the right foods can help you to lose weight, maintain a healthy weight, and even prevent chronic diseases. Here are some healthy food choices for weight loss:

- ***Fruits and Vegetables***: Fruits and vegetables are nutrient-dense and provide essential vitamins and minerals. They are also low in calories, which makes them perfect for weight loss. Choose from a variety of colourful produce such as apples, oranges, berries, carrots, spinach, and more.

- ***Whole Grains***: Whole grains are high in fibre and provide sustained energy throughout the day. Examples include oatmeal, brown rice, quinoa, and whole-wheat bread.

- ***Lean Protein:*** Lean protein helps to build and maintain muscle mass. Foods such as fish, poultry, eggs, and beans are excellent sources of lean protein.

- ***Healthy Fats:*** Healthy fats like avocados, nuts, and olive oil can help to keep you full and provide essential nutrients.

- ***Dairy:*** Low-fat dairy products provide essential vitamins and minerals. Choose from sources such as low-fat milk, yoghurt, and cheese.

By making healthy food choices, you can create a nutritious and balanced diet that will help you to reach your weight loss goals.

Healthy Fats

Healthy fats play an important role in weight loss and dieting. They provide energy, curb hunger, and help to keep your blood sugar levels stable. They also help to improve your digestion and absorption of nutrients. Healthy fats can be found in foods such as olive oil, nuts, and avocados.

Eating healthy fats can help to reduce your overall calorie intake. This is because they tend to be more filling than other types of food, so you will be less likely to overeat. Healthy fats also help to reduce inflammation in the body, which can help to reduce your risk of chronic diseases such as heart disease and diabetes.

Healthy fats also help to increase your metabolism, which can help to burn more calories. This can help to accelerate weight loss. Additionally, healthy fats can help to reduce your risk of developing certain medical conditions such as high cholesterol.

Including healthy fats in your diet is an important part of weight loss and dieting. They can help to reduce your calorie intake, improve your digestion, and reduce your risk of certain medical conditions. However, it is important to remember that healthy fats should be consumed in moderation. Too much of any type of fat can be unhealthy.

Don't forget to always consult your doctor before making any changes to your diet.

Lean Proteins

Lean proteins are an essential part of any weight loss and dieting plan. Lean proteins are typically low in fat and calories while providing a high-quality source of essential nutrients. Not only do lean proteins promote weight loss, but they also help to maintain muscle mass, which is important for overall health.

Lean proteins can help to reduce hunger and cravings, as they are digested slowly and keep you feeling fuller for longer. This can help to reduce overall calorie intake, which is important for weight loss. Lean proteins also help to burn calories, as the body needs more energy to digest them.

In addition to weight loss, lean proteins are also beneficial for overall health. They are high in essential nutrients such as iron, zinc, and B vitamins which are important for energy, metabolism, and cell repair. Lean proteins also contain essential fatty acids that are important for heart health and brain functioning.

When choosing lean proteins, it is important to look for lean cuts of meat, fish, and poultry. Eggs, legumes, nuts, and seeds are also good sources of lean protein. It is important to remember that while lean proteins are beneficial for weight loss, they should be eaten in moderation, as some are high in saturated fat and cholesterol.

In conclusion, lean proteins are an essential part of any weight loss and dieting plan. They are low in fat and calories while providing a high-quality source of essential nutrients that promote weight loss and overall health.

Example of lean protein

- ***Skinless Chicken Breast:*** Chicken breast is one of the leanest sources of protein and is packed with essential nutrients like B vitamins, iron, and zinc. It's also low in calories and fat, making it an ideal protein choice for weight loss and dieting.

- ***Turkey Breast:*** Like chicken breast, turkey breast is a lean source of protein that's low in fat and calories. It's also packed with essential nutrients like B vitamins, iron, and zinc.

- ***Fish:*** Fish is a great lean protein option for weight loss and dieting. It's high in omega-3 fatty acids, which have been linked to a reduced risk of certain types of cancer, heart disease, and stroke. It's also low in saturated fat and calories, making it an ideal choice for weight loss and dieting.

- ***Shellfish:*** Shellfish such as shrimp, lobster, and crab are lean sources of protein that are low in fat and calories. They are also packed with essential nutrients such as vitamin B12, zinc, and selenium.

- ***Eggs:*** Eggs are a great source of lean protein that can help you lose weight and maintain a healthy diet. They are also packed with essential nutrients such as vitamin B12, vitamin D, and lutein.

- ***Tofu:*** Tofu is a great plant-based source of lean protein that is low in fat and calories. It's also packed with essential nutrients such as iron, calcium, and magnesium.

- ***Greek Yoghourt:*** Greek yoghourt is a great source of lean protein that is low in fat and calories. It's also packed with essential nutrients such as calcium, potassium, and live active cultures.

- ***Nuts and Seeds:*** Nuts and seeds are great sources of lean protein that are low in fat and calories. They are also packed with essential nutrients such as magnesium, phosphorus, and zinc.

- ***Lentils:*** Lentils are a great source of lean protein that is low in fat and calories. They are also packed with essential nutrients such as folate, iron, and fibre.

- ***Edamame:*** Edamame is a great source of lean protein that is low in fat and calories. It's also packed with essential nutrients such as vitamin K, folate, and fibre.

Complex Carbohydrates

Complex carbohydrates are a type of carbohydrate that provide essential vitamins, minerals, and fibres needed for a healthy diet and weight loss. Complex carbohydrates are found in foods such as whole grains, vegetables, and legumes. These carbohydrates are broken down more slowly than simple carbohydrates and provide a steady source of energy throughout the day.

Eating complex carbohydrates can help with weight loss because they are low in calories and high in fibre, which can help you feel fuller for longer and reduce cravings. They also provide essential vitamins and minerals that can help improve overall health and energy levels. Additionally, complex carbohydrates can help stabilise blood sugar levels, which can help prevent overeating and energy crashes throughout the day.

Eating complex carbohydrates as part of a healthy diet can also help with weight loss by providing the body with essential nutrients. Eating complex carbohydrates can help keep the body fueled and energised, which can help with maintaining an active lifestyle and burning more calories. Additionally, complex carbohydrates can help keep the digestive system functioning properly, which can help improve overall health and weight loss.

Overall, complex carbohydrates are an important part of a healthy diet and weight loss plan. They provide essential vitamins, minerals, and fibres needed for a healthy diet, help stabilise blood sugar levels, and provide the body with energy to maintain an active lifestyle. Eating complex carbohydrates can help with weight loss and overall health.

Example of complex carbohydrate

- **Quinoa:** This nutrient-packed grain is high in fibre, protein, and complex carbohydrates, making it an ideal choice for weight loss and dieting.

- **Oats:** Oats are a rich source of complex carbohydrates, and they contain important nutrients like iron and B vitamins.

- **Sweet Potatoes:** Sweet potatoes are an excellent source of complex carbohydrates and they contain a host of vitamins and minerals.

- **Whole Wheat Bread:** Whole wheat bread contains complex carbohydrates, fibre, and other important nutrients.

- ***Brown Rice:*** Brown rice is a great source of complex carbohydrates and is low in fat and calories.

- ***Legumes:*** Beans, lentils, and peas are all great sources of complex carbohydrates and provide a healthy dose of protein and fibre.

- ***Barley:*** Barley is a complex carbohydrate-rich grain that is high in fibre and B vitamins.

- ***Whole Grain Pasta:****whole-grain pasta is* a great way to get complex carbohydrates, fibre, and protein.

- ***Bulgur:*** Bulgur is a type of wheat that is full of complex carbohydrates and other important nutrients.

- ***Buckwheat:*** Buckwheat is an excellent source of complex carbohydrates and is high in fibre and protein.

Chapter 3

Healthy Snacks

Healthy snacks can be a great way to stay on track with a weight-loss diet. Not only do snacks help keep hunger at bay between meals, but they can also provide important nutrients to help with the weight loss process.

When looking for healthy snacks, it's important to focus on those that are low in calories and high in nutrients. Here are some great snack ideas to help you stay on track with your weight loss goals:

- **Fruits and Vegetables:** Fresh fruits and vegetables are always a great snack as they are naturally low in calories and high in vitamins, minerals, and fibre. Have a handful of carrots, celery, cucumbers, or bell peppers for a nutrient-dense snack. You can also add some low-fat dip or hummus for extra flavour.

- **Nuts and Seeds:** Nuts and seeds are great sources of healthy fats and protein, which can help keep you feeling full. Go for raw, unsalted varieties and keep portions to 1/4 cup to keep calories in check.

- **Greek Yoghourt:** Greek yoghourt is a great snack because it's high in protein, which can help you feel fuller longer and keep cravings at bay. Look for low-fat, plain varieties and top them with some fresh fruit or nuts for extra flavour.

- **Air-popped Popcorn:** Air-popped popcorn is a great low-calorie snack. To make your own, just put some popcorn kernels in a brown paper bag and microwave for a few minutes. Top with some herbs and spices for extra flavour.

- **Whole-Grain Crackers:** Whole-grain crackers are a great alternative to chips and can be topped with healthy spreads like hummus or nut butter. Look for those that are low in sodium and added sugars.

Snacking can be a great tool for weight loss as long as you choose healthy snacks. Try to focus on those that are low in calories and high in nutrients to get the most out of your snacks.

But eating snacks should not replace meals. Be sure to focus on getting enough about Healthy Snacks for weight loss and dieting

Avoid Unhealthy snacks

When trying to lose weight, one of the most important things to keep in mind is avoiding unhealthy snacks. Unhealthy snacks can be a huge roadblock to reaching your weight loss goals. They are typically high in calories and fat and can contribute to weight gain and an unhealthy lifestyle.

The key to avoiding unhealthy snacks is to be mindful of what you are eating. Choose snacks that are healthy and nutritious, such as fruits, vegetables, nuts, and seeds. These snacks are packed with essential vitamins and minerals and can help keep you full longer. Try to avoid snacks that are high in sugar and saturated fat, such as candy, chips, and cookies.

In addition to avoiding unhealthy snacks, it is important to stay hydrated. Water is essential for weight loss and can help keep you feeling full and satisfied. at least eight glasses of water each day. If you find yourself craving snacks, try drinking a glass of water first. This can help curb your appetite and make it easier to resist unhealthy snacks.

Finally, it is important to plan when it comes to snacks. If you know you will be busy and on the go, make sure to pack some healthy snacks for the day. This can help you stay away from the unhealthy snacks that may be available.

Overall, avoiding unhealthy snacks is an important part of a successful weight loss and dieting plan. By being mindful of what you are eating and staying hydrated, you can help stay on track to achieving your goals.

Try to make healthy snacks a part of your routine and you will soon be on your way to a healthier lifestyle!

Nutrient-Dense Options

Nutrient-dense options for weight loss and dieting are important for anyone looking to shed pounds healthily. Nutrient-dense foods provide the body with essential vitamins, minerals, and other important nutrients that are necessary for optimal health.

Fruits and vegetables are some of the best nutrient-dense options for weight loss and dieting. They are packed with vitamins, minerals, fibre, antioxidants, and other essential nutrients. Fruits and vegetables are also low in calories, making them an excellent choice for anyone looking to lose weight. Eating a variety of fruits and vegetables is a great way to get a wide range of nutrients while also cutting back on calories.

Healthy proteins such as lean meats, fish, poultry, eggs, and legumes are also great nutrient-dense options for weight loss and dieting. They provide the body with energy, essential amino acids, and other important nutrients.

Protein is also filling, which can help to reduce cravings and keep you feeling full for longer. Eating a variety of healthy proteins can help to ensure that you are getting all the nutrients you need while also keeping calories low.

Whole grains are another great nutrient-dense option for weight loss and dieting. They provide the body with essential vitamins and minerals, fibre, and other important nutrients.

Whole grains also help to promote a feeling of fullness, which can help to reduce cravings and keep you from overeating.

Eating a variety of whole grains is a great way to get all the vitamins, minerals, and other nutrients you need while also keeping your calorie intake low.

 Finally, healthy fats such as avocados, nuts, and seeds are great nutrient-dense options for weight loss and dieting. They provide the body with essential fatty acids, fibre, and other important nutrients.

Healthy fats are also filling and can help to keep you feeling full for longer. Eating a variety of healthy fats is a great way to get all the nutrients you need while also keeping your calorie intake low.

By incorporating a variety of nutrient-dense options into your diet, you can ensure that you are getting all the essential vitamins, minerals, and other important nutrients your body needs while also keeping your calorie intake low. This will help to support your weight loss efforts and promote overall health.

Remember, nutrition is key when it comes to weight loss and dieting. Eating a variety of nutrient-dense foods is the best way to ensure that you are getting all the essential nutrients your body needs while also keeping your calorie intake low.

Chapter 4

Supplements

Weight loss supplements are popular among those looking to achieve a healthy body weight and improve their overall health. They are widely available in both natural and synthetic forms and can be used either as standalone products or in combination with a healthy diet and exercise plan.

Natural weight loss supplements are generally derived from plants and herbs and may contain vitamins, minerals, and other nutrients that can help to boost metabolism and reduce appetite.

These products may work by increasing thermogenesis, which is the body's ability to burn calories, or by reducing the absorption of fat and carbohydrates from the diet.

Some of the most popular natural weight loss supplements include green tea extract, garcinia Cambogia, and curcumin.

Synthetic weight loss supplements are typically created in a laboratory and are designed to mimic the effects of natural weight loss supplements. These products usually contain stimulants such as caffeine, guarana, and ephedra, which can increase energy levels and boost metabolism.

However, the use of synthetic weight loss supplements can be associated with several potential side effects, including insomnia, jitteriness, and an increased heart rate.

In addition to these weight loss supplements, several dieting and lifestyle plans can help to encourage healthy weight loss. These plans typically involve eating a balanced diet, reducing calorie intake, and increasing physical activity. They may also include the use of meal replacement shakes and bars, as well as supplements such as fibre and probiotics.

Weight loss supplements can be an effective way to jumpstart a weight loss program, but they should not be used as a replacement for a healthy diet and lifestyle. It is important to consult with a healthcare professional before beginning any weight loss or diet plan

Types of Supplements
1. **Protein Supplements:** Protein supplements are an excellent way to increase your protein intake, which can help with weight loss and dieting. Protein can help to build muscle and burn fat and is an essential nutrient for healthy weight loss. There are many different types of protein supplements, including powders, bars, and liquids.

2.**Fibre Supplements:** Fibre is an important part of any diet, and can help to reduce cravings and keep you feeling full for longer. Fibre supplements can come in the form of powders, capsules, and bars, and can help to increase your fibre intake without having to eat high-fibre foods.

3.**Herbal Supplements:** Herbal supplements can be a great addition to a healthy diet and can help to support weight loss. Some herbs that are believed to help with weight loss include green tea, garcinia Cambogia, and hoodia.

4.**Vitamins and Minerals:** Vitamins and minerals are essential for optimal health, and can help to support healthy weight loss. There are a variety of supplements that contain a variety of vitamins and minerals that can help to support healthy weight loss.

5.**Omega-3 Fatty Acids:** Omega-3 fatty acids are essential fatty acids that can help to support weight loss and dieting. They can be found in fish oil supplements, which can help to reduce inflammation, regulate metabolism, and support healthy weight loss.

These are just a few of the many types of supplements that can help to support healthy weight loss and dieting. It is important to consult with a healthcare professional before starting any supplement to ensure that it is appropriate for your individual needs.

When to Use Supplements

When it comes to weight loss and dieting, supplements can be an important tool in achieving your desired results. To get the most out of supplements, it is important to understand when they should be used and in what amount.

The best time to use supplements for weight loss and dieting is when you are trying to lose weight. Supplements can provide essential nutrients that your body needs to help with weight loss, such as vitamins, minerals, amino acids, and other beneficial compounds. Supplements can also help to boost your metabolism, which can help you burn more calories and lose weight faster.

When using supplements for weight loss and dieting, it is important to remember that they should never be used as a substitute for a well-balanced diet. Supplements should be used in conjunction with a healthy diet and exercise regimen. It is also important to make sure that you are getting enough essential nutrients from your diet so that your body can function properly.

When it comes to the number of supplements you should take, it is best to consult with your healthcare provider to determine the right amount for you. Supplements are not regulated by the FDA, so it is important to make sure you are taking the right amount for your needs.

Additionally, it is important to note that while supplements can help you reach your weight loss and dieting goals, they will not work if you do not make changes to your lifestyle.

In conclusion, supplements can be an important tool in helping you achieve your weight loss and dieting goals. However, it is important to remember that they should never be used as a substitute for a healthy diet and exercise regimen. Additionally, it is important to consult with your healthcare provider to determine the right amount of supplements for you.

These are just a few of the many types of supplements that can help to support healthy weight loss and dieting. It is important to consult with a healthcare professional before starting any supplement to ensure that it is appropriate for your individual needs.

Chapter 5

Keeping a Food Journal

A food journal is a great tool for tracking what you eat and managing your weight. Keeping an up-to-date food journal can help you identify patterns in your eating habits so that you can make informed changes to your diet and lifestyle.

When you start a food journal, you should include details such as what you ate, when you ate, how much you ate, where you ate, and how you felt before and after you ate. This will help you to identify potential triggers for overeating, such as boredom or stress. You may also want to track your physical activity and water intake in your journal.

You may find that keeping a food journal helps you to become more mindful of what you are eating. By writing down what you eat and how you feel before and after eating, you can begin to recognize patterns or habits that may be contributing to weight gain or unhealthy eating.

The key to keeping an up-to-date food journal is consistency. It's important to write down everything you eat, no matter how small, so that you can get a true picture of your eating habits. You should also make sure to update your journal regularly so that you can track changes over time.

By keeping an up-to-date food journal, you can gain insight into your eating habits and make changes that will help you reach your weight loss and dieting goals.

Chapter 6

30 days Meal Plan

Day One

Breakfast
Overnight oats with banana and almond butter.

Overnight oats are a great way to start the day with a delicious and nutritious breakfast. This overnight oats with banana and almond butter recipe is a great way to enjoy oats that are both tasty and filling.

1. Start by combining ½ cup of old-fashioned rolled oats with 1 cup of your favourite milk.

2. Add a pinch of salt and like maple syrup to taste.

3. Mix everything and let sit in the refrigerator overnight.

4. In the morning, top with ½ of a sliced banana and 1 tablespoon of almond butter.

5. Enjoy your overnight oats with banana and almond butter!

You can also mix in other ingredients like chia seeds, nuts, and dried fruit for added flavour and nutrition.

This overnight oats recipe makes a great meal for any time of the day and can be enjoyed hot or cold. Enjoy! Preparation time: 10 minutes

Snack
Apple slices with a tablespoon of peanut butter

Gather the ingredients: two apples, one tablespoon of creamy peanut butter, a knife, and a cutting board.

2. Wash the apples and dry them with a paper towel.

3. Cut the apples into thin slices.

4. Spread the peanut butter on each apple slice.

5. Enjoy your healthy snack! Preparation time: 5 minutes

Lunch
Grilled chicken breast with brown rice and steamed broccoli.

Ingredients:
-2 boneless, skinless chicken breasts
-1/2 cup uncooked brown rice
-1 head of fresh broccoli
-1 tablespoon olive oil
-Salt and pepper to taste

Instructions:
1. Preheat your grill to medium-high heat.

2. Place the chicken breasts onto a plate, season with salt and pepper, and brush each side lightly with olive oil.

3. Place the chicken onto the preheated grill and cook for 4 minutes per side, or until the internal temperature reaches 165°F.

4. While the chicken is cooking, prepare the brown rice according to the package instructions.

5. Clean and trim the broccoli and place it in a steamer basket. Steam the broccoli until it's just tender, about 8 minutes.

6. Serve the grilled chicken breasts with brown rice and steamed broccoli. Enjoy! Preparation time: 15 minutes

Snack
Celery sticks with hummus.

1. Begin by washing and cutting the celery into sticks. Cut the celery into pieces that are roughly 4-5 inches long.

2. Prep the hummus. You can either buy store-bought hummus or you can make your own by blending cooked chickpeas, tahini, garlic, lemon juice, and olive oil.

3. Place the celery sticks in a bowl and spread them out.

4. Spread the hummus onto the celery sticks. You can either use a spoon or a knife to do this.

5. Sprinkle some salt and pepper onto the hummus-covered celery sticks, if desired.

6. Serve the celery sticks with hummus and enjoy!
Preparation time: 5 minutes

Dinner
Baked salmon with quinoa and roasted Brussels sprouts

Ingredients:

-4 6-ounce salmon fillets
-1 cup uncooked quinoa
-2 tablespoons olive oil

-1/2 teaspoon salt
-1/4 teaspoon black pepper
-1/2 teaspoon dried oregano
-1/4 teaspoon garlic powder
-1/4 teaspoon paprika
-1/4 teaspoon cumin
-1/2 lemon, sliced
-1/2 pound Brussels sprouts, trimmed and halved

Instructions:

1. Preheat the oven to 375 degrees F. Lightly grease a baking sheet.

2. In a medium saucepan, add quinoa and 2 cups of water. Bring to a boil, reduce heat to low, and simmer for 15 minutes, or until the quinoa is cooked.

3. In a small bowl, combine the olive oil, salt, pepper, oregano, garlic powder, paprika, and cumin.

4. Place the salmon fillets on the prepared baking sheet. Brush each fillet with the olive oil mixture and top with lemon slices.

5. In a separate bowl, toss the Brussels sprouts with the remaining olive oil mixture. Arrange the Brussels sprouts around the salmon.

6. Bake for 20 minutes, or until the salmon is cooked through and the Brussels sprouts are tender.

7. Serve the salmon with the quinoa and roasted Brussels sprouts. Enjoy!
Preparation time: 20 minutes

Day two

Breakfast
Avocado toast with poached eggs.

Avocado toast with poached eggs is a delicious and easy breakfast. Here's how to make it:

1. Begin by preparing the ingredients. Slice the avocado into thin slices and set aside. Heat a pot of water on the stove until it reaches a gentle simmer.

2. Toast some bread in a toaster or then.

3 thread is a generous layer of mashed avocado onto each slice.

4. Crack two eggs into a small bowl and gently pour them into the simmering water. Poach them for about 3 minutes until the whites are set.

5. Carefully remove the eggs from the water using a slotted spoon.

6. Place the poached eggs on top of the avocado toast and season with salt and pepper.

7. Enjoy your avocado toast with poached eggs!

Preparation time: 10 minutes

Snack
Handful of nuts.

Making a handful of nuts is a great way to enjoy a healthy snack. The best part is that you can customise your handful of nuts to include the flavours and textures that you prefer! Here's a guide on how to make a flavorful handful of nuts:

1. Gather your ingredients. You'll need a variety of nuts such as almonds, walnuts, cashews, and pecans. You can also add seeds such as pumpkin and sunflower.

2. Toast the nuts. Toasting the nuts adds an extra layer of flavour and crunch. Preheat the oven to 350°F, spread the nuts on a baking sheet, and bake for 8-10 minutes.

3. Season the nuts. Once the nuts are toasted, sprinkle them with a pinch of salt and your favourite spices such as cinnamon, cumin, or chilli powder.

4. Enjoy your handful of nuts. Place the seasoned nuts in a bowl and enjoy them as a snack! You can also add them to salads, pasta, and other dishes for added crunch and flavour.
Preparation time: 5 minutes

Lunch

Kale salad with grilled chicken, tomatoes, and balsamic vinaigrette.

1. Prepare the salad and vinaigrette ingredients first. Remove any woody centre stems after washing the kale. Cut the kale into bite-sized pieces, then add it to a big bowl. Add the tomato slices to the bowl. Season the chicken with salt and pepper after slicing it into thin pieces.

2. To make the vinaigrette, whisk together the balsamic vinegar, olive oil, garlic, honey, salt, and pepper in a small bowl.

3. Turn the heat to medium-high on a grill or grill pan. The chicken should be cooked through after grilling the strips for 4–5 minutes on each side.

4. Remove the chicken from the grill and add to the bowl with the kale and tomatoes. Drizzle the dressing over the top and toss to combine.

5. Serve the kale salad with grilled chicken, tomatoes, and balsamic vinaigrette. Enjoy!

Preparation time: 15 minutes

Baked cod with steamed cauliflower and lemon.

1. Preheat the oven to 375°F.

2. Line a baking sheet with parchment paper.

3. Place the cod fillets on the parchment paper and season with salt, pepper, and lemon juice.

4. Bake in the preheated oven for 12-15 minutes, or until the cod is cooked through.

5. While the cod is baking, steam the cauliflower florets in a steamer basket over boiling water. Cook for 5-7 minutes, or until tender.

6. Place the cooked cauliflower in a bowl and toss it with olive oil, salt, pepper, and lemon juice.

7. When the cod is done, remove it from the oven and let cool slightly.

8. Serve the cod with steamed cauliflower and a wedge of lemon. Enjoy!
Preparation time: 15 minutes

Day Three

Scrambled egg whites with spinach and mushrooms.

Ingredients:

-1/2 cup egg whites
-2 tablespoons diced mushrooms
-2 tablespoons chopped fresh spinach
-1 tablespoon olive oil
-Salt and pepper to taste

Instructions:

1. Heat the olive oil in a skillet over medium heat.

2. Add the mushrooms and sauté for 3-4 minutes until lightly browned.

3. Add the spinach and sauté for another 1-2 minutes until the spinach is wilted.

4. Pour in the egg whites and season with salt and pepper to taste.

5. Using a spatula, mix the eggs and vegetables.

6. Cook for about 3-4 minutes, stirring occasionally, until the eggs are cooked through.

7. Serve the scrambled egg whites with spinach and mushrooms hot. Enjoy!
Preparation time: 10 minutes

Snack
Celery sticks with almond butter.

Celery sticks with almond butter make a delicious and nutritious snack that's easy to prepare. To make them, you'll need a few basic ingredients: celery, almond butter, and your favourite toppings. Here's how to make it:

1. Wash and cut the celery into sticks.

2. Spread a generous amount of almond butter on each celery stick.

3. Sprinkle your favourite toppings over the almond butter, such as raisins, sunflower seeds, or chopped nuts.

4. Enjoy your healthy snack!

You can also make this snack more interesting by substituting peanut butter for almond butter. You can also add other ingredients, like cream cheese or hummus, to make different flavour combinations. Celery sticks with almond butter are a great way to get your daily dose of nutrients while satisfying your cravings for something delicious.

Preparation time: 5 minutes

Turkey wrap with tomatoes, lettuce, and hummus

Making a turkey wrap with tomatoes, lettuce, and hummus is a delicious and healthy lunch option. Here are the steps to make the wrap:

1. Gather the ingredients. You will need 2 large tortillas, turkey slices (about 4-5 ounces), 1 cup of lettuce, 1 tomato sliced into thin wedges, and 2 tablespoons of hummus.

2. Place the tortillas on a flat surface. Spread the hummus on one side of each tortilla.

3. Place the turkey slices in the centre of each tortilla.

4. Top with lettuce and tomatoes.

5. Roll up the tortilla, making sure to tuck it in the sides.

6. Cut the wrap into two pieces and enjoy!

Making a turkey wrap with tomatoes, lettuce, and hummus is a quick and easy way to have a tasty lunch. It's also a great way to get some protein and vegetables in your diet. Enjoy!

Preparation time: 10 minutes

Whole wheat crackers with cottage cheese.

Ingredients:

- 1 cup whole wheat flour
- 2 tablespoons olive oil
- 1/4 teaspoon salt
- 1/2 cup cottage cheese
- 2-3 tablespoons water

Instructions:

1. Preheat the oven to 375°F.

2. In a mixing bowl, combine flour, olive oil, and salt.

3. Add cottage cheese and combine with a wooden spoon.

4. Slowly add water until the dough forms a ball.

5. Place the dough on a lightly floured surface and roll out to 1/4 inch thick.

6. Cut out crackers with a cookie cutter.

7. Place the crackers on a lightly greased baking sheet.

8. Bake for 12-15 minutes or until golden brown.

9. Let cool before serving. Enjoy!

Preparation time: 5 minutes

Dinner:
Baked sweet potato with grilled shrimp and sautéed vegetables.

Ingredients:

-2 large sweet potatoes, scrubbed and pierced with a fork
-1 lb. shrimp, peeled and deveined
-1 red bell pepper, cored and diced
-1 onion, diced
-2 cloves garlic, minced
-1 tbsp. olive oil
-1 tsp. smoked paprika
-1 tsp. garlic powder
-Salt and pepper, to taste
-2 tbsp. fresh parsley, chopped

Instructions:

1. Preheat the oven to 400°F. Place sweet potatoes on a baking sheet and bake for 45 minutes, or until they are soft when pierced with a fork.

2. 2. In the meantime, warm the oil in a sizable skillet over medium-high heat. Add shrimp, bell pepper, onion, and garlic and cook until shrimp is cooked through and vegetables are tender for about 5 minutes.

3. Add smoked paprika, garlic powder, salt, and pepper to the skillet and cook for another minute.

4. Serve sweet potatoes with grilled shrimp and sautéed vegetables, garnished with parsley. Enjoy!

Preparation time: 20 minutes

Day Four

Breakfast
Smoothie bowl with banana, almond milk, and chia seeds.

To make a smoothie bowl with banana, almond milk, and chia seeds, you will need the following ingredients:

-1 banana, peeled and sliced into 1-inch chunks
-1 cup almond milk
-2 tablespoons chia seeds
-Optional: 1 tablespoon honey or maple syrup for added sweetness

Instructions:

1. Place the banana slices in a blender and blend until creamy.

2. Add the almond milk and blend until combined.

3. Add the chia seeds and blend until everything is well combined.

4. If desired, add honey or maple syrup for added sweetness.

5. Pour the mixture into a bowl and top with desired toppings, such as fresh fruit, nuts, and/or granola.

6. Enjoy your delicious, nutrient-packed smoothie bowl!

Preparation time: 10 minutes

Snack

Apple slices with peanut butter

Ingredients:

-2 Large Apples

-1/4 Cup of Natural Peanut Butter

-1/4 Cup of Dried Fruit (optional)

Instructions:

1. Begin by washing the apples and then slicing each one into 8-12 thin slices.

2. Place the apple slices on a plate.

3. Spread a thin layer of peanut butter on each apple slice.

4. Sprinkle the dried fruit (optional) on top of each slice.

5. Enjoy your delicious and healthy snack!

Preparation time: 5 minutes

Grilled chicken with quinoa and roasted vegetables.

Ingredients

- 1 lb boneless, skinless chicken breasts
- 1 cup quinoa
- 2 tablespoons olive oil
- 1 teaspoon garlic powder
- 1 teaspoon smoked paprika
- Salt and pepper
- 2 cups of your favourite roasted vegetables

Instructions

1. Preheat your oven to 375°F and line a baking sheet with parchment paper.

2. In a medium bowl, combine the quinoa with 1 tablespoon of olive oil, garlic powder, smoked paprika, salt, and pepper. Spread the quinoa onto the prepared baking sheet and bake for 20 minutes.

3. Meanwhile, season the chicken breasts with salt and pepper and heat a large skillet over medium-high heat. Add 1 tablespoon of olive oil to the skillet and cook the chicken breasts until golden and cooked through, about 5-7 minutes per side.

4. Remove the quinoa from the oven and add the roasted vegetables to the baking sheet. Return to the oven and bake for an additional 15 minutes.

5. Serve the roasted vegetables and quinoa with the grilled chicken. Enjoy!

Preparation time: 15 minutes

Snack
Celery sticks with hummus.

To make celery sticks with hummus, you will need celery, hummus, and your favourite veggies.

1. Begin by washing and cutting the celery into 3- to 4-inch sticks.

2. Place the celery sticks on a plate.

3. Prepare your favourite hummus recipe. If you don't have a recipe, you can find many online or in cookbooks.

4. Spread the hummus on the celery sticks.

5. Top the celery sticks with your favourite vegetables. Some ideas are tomatoes, cucumbers, bell peppers, or olives.

6. Serve the celery sticks with hummus and vegetables. Enjoy!

Preparation time: 5 minutes

Dinner
Baked salmon with sweet potato and steamed broccoli.

Ingredients:
- 1 salmon fillet
- 1 sweet potato
- 2 handfuls of broccoli

Instructions:
1. Preheat the oven to 375°F.
2. Peel and chop the sweet potato into 1-inch cubes and spread them onto a baking sheet. Drizzle with olive oil and sprinkle with salt and pepper.
3. Place the salmon fillet on a separate baking sheet and season with salt and pepper.
4. Bake the sweet potato and salmon for about 20 minutes, or until the sweet potato is fork-tender and the salmon is cooked through.
5. While the salmon and sweet potato are baking, steam the broccoli for about 5 minutes.
6. Serve the salmon, sweet potato, and steamed broccoli together. Enjoy!
Preparation time: 20 minutes

Day Five

Breakfast
Oatmeal with fresh fruit and nuts.

Oatmeal with fresh fruit and nuts is a healthy and delicious breakfast option for those looking to lose weight or who are following a diet. To make oatmeal with fresh fruit and nuts, you will need:

-1 cup of old-fashioned oats
-2 cups of water
-1/2 cup of fresh fruit (berries, chopped apples, bananas, etc.)
-1/4 cup of nuts (almonds, walnuts, pecans, etc.)
-1/4 teaspoon of ground cinnamon
-1 tablespoon of honey

Step 1: Boil the water in a medium-sized pot.

Step 2: Once boiling, add the oats and stir.

Step 3: Reduce the heat to low and allow the oats to simmer for about 5 minutes, stirring occasionally.

Step 4: Once the oats are cooked, add the fresh fruit, nuts, and cinnamon.

Step 5: Stir to combine and simmer for an additional 5 minutes.

Step 6: Add the honey or maple syrup (optional) to sweeten.

Step 7: Serve the oatmeal with fresh fruit and nuts in individual bowls. Enjoy!

Oatmeal with fresh fruit and nuts is a nutritious and filling breakfast option that can help you reach your weight loss and dieting goals. It is quick and easy to make and will keep you feeling full until lunchtime. Enjoy!

Preparation time: 10 minutes

Snack
A handful of nuts.

Cooking handfuls of nuts for weight loss and dieting can be a great way to get the necessary nutrition while sticking to a calorie-controlled diet. Nuts are packed with essential nutrients and healthy fats, making them a great snack for those looking to lose weight. Here are some tips to make sure your handfuls of nuts are cooked just right for optimal weight loss and dieting.

1. **Choose the Right Nuts:** When it comes to weight loss and dieting, the type of nuts you choose is important. Nuts such as almonds, walnuts, and cashews

are lower in calories and fat than some other varieties and are a good choice for weight loss.

2. **Roast Nuts in the Oven:** Roasting nuts will bring out their natural flavour and make them more enjoyable to eat. Preheat the oven to 350° Fahrenheit and spread the nuts out on a baking sheet. Roast for 10-15 minutes, stirring occasionally to ensure they don't burn.

3. **Season and Add Flavor:** Once roasted, you can add flavour to your nuts with a variety of seasonings. A pinch of salt, pepper, garlic powder, or your favourite herbs or spices can all add flavour without compromising the health benefits of the nuts.

4. **Portion Control:** It's important to practise portion control when eating nuts for weight loss. A good rule of thumb is to have a handful of nuts (about 1/4 cup) as a snack. This way, you can still enjoy the health benefits of nuts without overdoing them.

By following these simple tips, you can make sure your handfuls of nuts are cooked to perfection and help you reach your weight loss goals. Bon appetit!
Preparation time: 5 minutes

Lunch
Lentil soup with a side of whole wheat toast.

Lentil soup is an ideal meal for weight loss and dieting. It is low in calories, high in protein and fibre, and also provides essential vitamins and minerals. Here is a recipe for a delicious lentil soup with a side of whole wheat toast that will help you reach your weight loss and dieting goals.

To begin, you'll need 1 cup of lentils, 1 can of diced tomatoes, and 2 cups of vegetable broth. First, heat a large pot over medium heat and add a tablespoon of olive oil. Add the lentils and stir until they're lightly toasted. Then add the tomatoes, broth, and any desired seasonings. Bring the soup to a boil, reduce heat, and simmer for about 35 minutes or until the lentils are tender.

While the soup is simmering, prepare the toast. Preheat the oven to 350°F. Slice a whole wheat loaf of bread into 8 slices, and spread 1 teaspoon of butter or margarine onto each slice. Place the slices on a baking sheet, and bake for 8-10 minutes or until lightly browned.

Once the soup and toast are ready, serve the soup in a bowl with a side of toast. Enjoy
 Preparation time: 35 minutes

Yoghurt with berries.

Cooking yoghurt with berries for weight loss and dieting is an easy, healthy way to reduce your calorie intake. You can make a delicious, nutritious meal by combining plain or flavoured yoghurts with a variety of fresh or frozen berries. This can be a great meal for breakfast, lunch, or dinner and is a great way to add some extra nutrition to your diet.

To make this meal, start by selecting your yoghurt. You can choose plain yoghurt or flavoured yoghurts, depending on your preference. For extra nutritional value, choose yoghurt that is high in protein and low in sugar. Once you have your yoghurt, add in your choice of berries. You can opt for fresh or frozen berries, depending on what is available.

After you have chosen your yoghurt and berries, mix them in a bowl. If you are using frozen berries, let them thaw first so that the yoghurt and berries can be properly mixed. Once the mixture is ready, pour it into a container and place it in the refrigerator. This can be taken cold or hot.

Eating yoghurt with berries for weight loss and dieting is an easy way to reduce your calorie intake without sacrificing taste. The combination of yoghourt and berries offers a variety of nutrients

Preparation time: 5 minutes

Dinner
Baked cod with roasted Brussels sprouts and lemon.

Ingredients:

- 4 cod fillets
- 2 tablespoons olive oil
- Salt and pepper to taste
- 2 cups Brussels sprouts, halved
- 2 cloves garlic, minced
- 1 lemon, cut into wedges

Instructions:

1. Preheat the oven to 375°F.

2. Put the cod fillets in a baking dish suitable for the oven. Add some salt and pepper, then sprinkle the remaining olive oil over everything.

3. Surround the cod with Brussels sprouts and garlic. Add some salt and pepper, then sprinkle the remaining olive oil over everything.

4. Place the lemon wedges around the cod and vegetables.

5. Bake for 20 minutes or until the cod is cooked through and the Brussels sprouts are tender.

6. Serve with a lemon wedge and enjoy!
Preparation time: 20 minutes

Day 6

Breakfast

Avocado toast with poached eggs.

Avocado Toast with Poached Eggs is a delicious and healthy dish that can help you with weight loss and dieting. This meal is packed with protein, fibre, healthy fats, and vitamins and minerals that will help you feel full and satisfied for longer. Here's how to make it:

Ingredients:

• 2 slices of whole wheat toast
2 eggs
• 2 tablespoons of olive oil
• 1 ripe avocado, diced
• Salt and pepper, to taste
• Optional: red pepper flakes, fresh herbs, garlic powder

Instructions:

1. Begin by preparing your poached eggs. To do this, fill a medium-sized pot with enough water to cover the eggs, and bring it to a boil. Once boiling, reduce the heat to medium-low and add the eggs. Simmer for 4-5 minutes, or until the egg whites are just set.

2. Meanwhile, lightly toast the bread. Once toasted, spread the avocado on top of the toast.

3. Once the eggs are done, carefully remove them from the pot and place them on top of the avocado-topped toast. Sprinkle with salt, pepper, and any other desired seasonings.

4. Drizzle with olive oil and serve.

Enjoy your Avocado Toast with Poached Eggs! Not only is this dish delicious, but it's also a healthy and satisfying meal that can help you with weight loss and dieting.
 Preparation time: 10 minutes

Snack
Apple slices with peanut butter.

Cooking apple slices with peanut butter is a great way to add a nutritious snack to your weight loss and dieting plan. Here is how you can make this delicious treat:

First, take an apple and slice it into thin pieces. Place the slices on a plate and spread a thin layer of peanut butter onto each piece. Make sure to use an all-natural, unsweetened variety.

Next, place the apple slices in the oven or toaster oven and cook them at 350 degrees Fahrenheit for 10-15 minutes or until the apples are soft and the peanut butter is melted.

Once the apples are cooked, take them out of the oven and let them cool. Then, enjoy your apple slices with peanut butter!

This snack is perfect for a quick, healthy, and tasty treat when you're trying to lose weight. The apple slices provide fibre, vitamins, and minerals, while the peanut butter adds protein and healthy fats to keep you full. Plus, the peanut butter adds a delicious flavour to the apples. Enjoy!

Preparation time: 5 minutes

Lunch

Greek salad with grilled chicken, feta cheese, and olives.

Greek Salad with Grilled Chicken, Feta Cheese, and Olives for Weight Loss and Dieting

Ingredients:

-2 cups romaine lettuce, chopped
-1/2 cup cucumber, chopped
-1 cup cherry tomatoes, halved
-1/4 cup red onion, diced
-1/4 cup Kalamata olives, pitted and halved
-1/4 cup feta cheese, crumbled
-1 boneless, skinless chicken breast, grilled
-2 tablespoons extra-virgin olive oil
-1 tablespoon red wine vinegar
-1 teaspoon dried oregano
-Salt and pepper, to taste

Instructions:

1. Preheat the grill to medium-high heat.

2. Rub the chicken breast with olive oil and season with salt and pepper.

3. Grill the chicken for 6-7 minutes per side, or until cooked through. Remove from the grill and set aside.

4. In a large bowl, combine the lettuce, cucumber, tomatoes, red onion, olives, and feta cheese.

5. Slice the grilled chicken and add to the salad.

6. In a small bowl, whisk together the olive oil, red wine vinegar, oregano, and salt and pepper.

7. Drizzle the dressing over the salad and toss to combine.

8. Serve the salad immediately and enjoy!
 Preparation time: 15 minutes

Snack
Celery sticks with almond butter.

Ingredients:

- 2 celery sticks

- 2 tablespoons of almond butter

- Salt and pepper, to taste

Instructions:

1. Wash the celery sticks and cut them into 3-4 inch pieces.

2. Spread the almond butter evenly over the celery sticks.

3. Sprinkle salt and pepper, to taste.

4. Enjoy your healthy snack!

This is a great snack for weight loss and dieting because it is low in calories and high in fibre. The almond butter adds healthy fats and protein to keep you full, while the celery sticks provide a crunchy texture. Enjoy your snack!
Preparation time: 5 minutes

Dinner
Baked sweet potato with grilled shrimp and steamed vegetables.

Ingredients:

- 1 sweet potato
- 1 pound of shrimp, peeled and deveined
- 2 cups of chopped vegetables (such as carrots, bell peppers, broccoli, and cauliflower)
- 2 tablespoons olive oil
- Salt and pepper to taste

Instructions:

1. Preheat the oven to 400°F.

2. Pierce the sweet potato with a fork and place it on a baking sheet. Bake for about 40 minutes, or until the sweet potato is tender when poked with a fork.

3. Heat a large skillet over medium-high heat. Add the olive oil, then add the shrimp. Season with salt and pepper and cook for about 3 minutes, or until shrimp is cooked through.

4. Add the chopped vegetables to the skillet and cook for an additional 3 minutes, stirring occasionally.

5. Slice the sweet potato in half and top it with the shrimp and vegetables. Serve warm. Enjoy!
Preparation time: 20 minutes

Day 7

Scrambled egg whites with spinach and mushrooms.

Ingredients:

-2 egg whites

-1 handful of fresh spinach

-1/4 cup mushrooms, sliced

-Salt and pepper, to taste

-1 teaspoon olive oil

Instructions:

1. Heat olive oil in a non-stick skillet over medium heat.

2. Add mushrooms and sauté until lightly browned and softened, about 5 minutes.

3. Add spinach and cook for another 2 minutes.

4. In a separate bowl, whisk together egg whites and season with salt and pepper.

5. Pour egg whites into the skillet and stir until eggs are cooked through for about 2 minutes.

6. Serve warm. Enjoy!
Preparation time: 10 minutes

Handful of nuts.

A handful of nuts is a great snack for weight loss and dieting. Not only are they full of healthy fats and protein, but they also provide essential vitamins and minerals. Here's how to make a handful of nuts for weight loss and dieting:

1. Choose your nuts. There are many different types of nuts to choose from, such as almonds, walnuts, cashews, and pistachios. Choose whichever type you prefer or mix and match.

2. Measure out a handful of nuts. A single serving of nuts is typically one ounce or about two tablespoons. This is roughly equivalent to one handful.

3. Roast the nuts. Roasting your nuts can make them more flavorful and crunchy. Preheat your oven to 350°F and spread a single layer of nuts on a baking sheet lined with parchment paper. Bake for 10-15 minutes, stirring once or twice, until golden and fragrant.

4. Add some flavour. Add a pinch of salt or a sprinkle of your favourite spices such as cinnamon, nutmeg, or allspice.

5. Enjoy your healthy snack. Eat your roasted nuts as a snack or sprinkle them over your favourite salads or yoghurt. They make a great addition to any meal!

Making a handful of nuts is an easy and healthy way to add a bit of crunch to your diet. Eating nuts regularly is linked to many health benefits, such as reducing the risk of heart disease and promoting weight loss. So, snack on a handful of nuts and enjoy the health benefits!
Preparation time: 5 minutes

Quinoa bowl with grilled chicken, tomatoes, and balsamic vinaigrette.

1. Begin by cooking the quinoa according to the package instructions.

2. While the quinoa is cooking, prepare the grilled chicken. Preheat the grill or a large skillet. Season the chicken with salt, pepper, and any other desired herbs and spices. Grill the chicken on both sides for about 5 minutes per side, or until cooked through.

3. Slice the tomatoes and set aside.

4. Make the balsamic vinaigrette by combining balsamic vinegar, olive oil, Dijon mustard, honey, garlic, salt, and pepper in a small bowl. Whisk until combined.

5. Once the quinoa is cooked, assemble the bowl. Add the quinoa to the bowl and top with the grilled chicken, tomatoes, and balsamic vinaigrette.

6. Enjoy! This quinoa bowl is a great meal for weight loss and dieting. It tastes great and is flavorful, light, and healthy.
Preparation time: 15 minutes

Snack
Whole wheat crackers with cottage cheese.

Making whole wheat crackers with cottage cheese for weight loss and dieting is a simple and delicious way to enjoy a healthy snack. Here are the steps to make this tasty treat:

1. 1. Turn the oven's temperature up to 350 degrees Fahrenheit.

2. In a medium-sized bowl, mix 1 cup of whole wheat flour, 1 teaspoon of baking powder, and ½ teaspoon of salt.

3. Add in 2 tablespoons of melted butter, and mix until combined.

4. In a separate bowl, mix 1 cup of cottage cheese, 1 egg, and 2 tablespoons of honey.

5. Add the wet ingredients to the dry ingredients, and stir until combined.

6. Use your hands to press the dough into a ball, and then roll it out on a lightly floured surface.

7. Cut the dough into small cracker-sized shapes, and place them on a baking sheet lined with parchment paper.

8. Bake for 12–15 minutes, or until the crackers are golden brown.

9. Let the crackers cool before serving. Enjoy!

These crackers are a great snack to eat while dieting and trying to lose weight. They are low in calories, but still provide a good source of protein and fibre. Enjoy this delicious treat as part of a balanced diet and lifestyle for the best results.
 Preparation time: 5 minutes

Baked salmon with quinoa and roasted Brussels sprouts.

Ingredients:

- 4 (6-ounce) salmon fillets
- 2 cups cooked quinoa
- 2 tablespoons olive oil
- 2 cloves garlic, minced
- 1 teaspoon Italian seasoning
- 1/4 teaspoon sea salt
- 2 cups Brussels sprouts, cut in half and trimmed
- 1 teaspoon freshly ground black pepper

Instructions:

1. Preheat the oven to 400°F.

2. Set the salmon fillets in a baking pan that is not too deep.

3. In a separate bowl, combine quinoa, olive oil, garlic, Italian seasoning, and sea salt. Mix until combined.

4. Spread the quinoa mixture evenly over the salmon.

5. Arrange the Brussels sprouts around the salmon. Sprinkle it with black pepper.

6. Bake for 15-20 minutes or until the salmon is cooked through and the Brussels sprouts are tender.

7. Serve and enjoy!

Preparation time: 20 minutes

Day 8

Overnight oats with banana and almond butter.

Overnight oats with banana and almond butter are a great way to get in healthy nutrition while on a weight loss and diet plan. This delicious meal is easy to make and can be prepared the night before so you can have a quick and nutritious breakfast the next day. Here's how to make it:

1. Start by combining 1/2 cup of rolled oats, 1/2 cup of almond milk, and 1/2 teaspoon of ground cinnamon in a bowl.

2. Mix the ingredients until the oats are fully coated in the almond milk and cinnamon.

3. Place the mixture in a sealable container or jar and leave it in the fridge overnight.

4. The next morning, take out your overnight oats and top them with 1/2 a banana, sliced, and 1 tablespoon of almond butter.

5. Enjoy your overnight oats with banana and almond butter as a healthy, delicious breakfast.

This nutritious and delicious breakfast is a great way to start your day when you're trying to lose weight and eat healthily. Oats are a great source of dietary fibre and protein, while almond butter and banana provide healthy fats and carbohydrates. Enjoy this meal as part of your weight loss and diet plan!

Preparation time: 10 minutes

Snack

Celery sticks with hummus.

Celery sticks with hummus are a great snack for weight loss and dieting. Not only is it easy to make, but it is also a nutritious snack that will help you stay full and energised throughout the day. Here's how to make it:

1. Start by washing and cutting your celery into sticks. Depending on your preference, cut them into desired sizes.

2. Place the celery sticks in a bowl and set aside.

3. In a separate bowl, mix one cup of plain hummus with two tablespoons of olive oil. You can also add other seasonings or spices to your hummus, such as garlic, lemon, or even chilli powder.

4. Dip the celery sticks into the hummus and enjoy!

Celery sticks with hummus are a great snack for weight loss and dieting because it's low in calories and high in fibre. The hummus adds a creamy and delicious flavour to the celery, and it's also a great source of protein. Enjoy this snack as a mid-morning snack or as a part of your lunch and dinner.

Preparation time: 5 minutes

Lunch
Kale salad with grilled chicken, tomatoes, and balsamic vinaigrette.

Making a Kale Salad with grilled chicken, tomatoes and balsamic vinaigrette is a great way to get a healthy and nutritious meal that is perfect for weight loss and dieting. Here are the steps to make this delicious and nutritious salad:

1. Begin by preparing the kale by removing the ribs and stems and cutting the leaves into thin strips. Place the kale in a large bowl and toss with a pinch of salt and pepper.

2. Next, heat a large skillet over medium-high heat and add a tablespoon of olive oil. Once the oil is hot, add the diced chicken and cook until it is browned and cooked through. Once the chicken is cooked, remove it from the heat and set aside.

3. To assemble the salad, add the kale to the bowl, followed by the grilled chicken, diced tomatoes, and balsamic vinaigrette. Mix everything, then add more salt and pepper to your taste.

4. Serve the salad immediately as a side dish or as a main course. Enjoy!

This Kale Salad with grilled chicken, tomatoes, and balsamic vinaigrette is a great way to get a healthy and nutritious meal that is perfect for weight loss and dieting. It is packed with protein, vitamins, and minerals, and the addition of the balsamic vinaigrette adds a delicious and tangy flavour that is sure to please. Enjoy!
 Preparation time: 15 minutes

Snack
Apple slices with a tablespoon of peanut butter.

Making apple slices with a tablespoon of peanut butter is a great way to incorporate a healthy snack into your weight loss and dieting plan. Here's how to do it:

1. Begin by washing and drying an apple of your choice.

2. Slice the apple into thin slices and place them on a plate.

3. Place a tablespoon of peanut butter in a small bowl and microwave it for 10-15 seconds until it's melted and spreadable.

4. Use a spoon to spread the melted peanut butter over the apple slices.

5. Enjoy your tasty snack!

This snack is a great option for those looking to lose weight or maintain a healthy diet. Apples contain fibre, vitamins, and minerals, while peanut butter is a good source of protein and healthy fats. Eating this snack regularly can help you feel fuller for longer and provide you with the nutrition your body needs.

Preparation time: 5 minutes

Dinner
Baked cod with steamed cauliflower and lemon.

Baked cod with steamed cauliflower and lemon is a healthy and delicious dish that is ideal for those looking to lose weight and maintain a healthy diet. This recipe is easy to make and provides a great source of lean protein and fibre.

Your oven should first be preheated to 375 degrees Fahrenheit.

Rinse and pat dry a cod fillet, then season with salt and pepper. Place the cod fillet on a parchment-lined baking sheet.

Steam a head of cauliflower until it is tender, about 5-7 minutes. Transfer the steamed cauliflower to a bowl, then season with salt and pepper.

Add fresh lemon juice and extra virgin olive oil.

Place the cod fillet and the cauliflower on the baking sheet and bake for about 15-20 minutes, or until the cod is cooked through.

Serve the baked cod with the steamed cauliflower and lemon for a healthy, delicious, and weight-loss-friendly meal. Enjoy!

This dish is low in fat and calories, yet high in fibre and protein. It is also a great source of healthy Omega-3 fatty acids. With its combination of flavours and nutrients, this dish is sure to help you reach your weight loss and dieting goals.

Preparation time: 15 minutes

Day 9

Breakfast: Smoothie bowl with banana, almond milk, and chia seeds.

Making a smoothie bowl with banana, almond milk, and chia seeds is an easy and delicious way to get a healthy start to your day. This smoothie bowl is ideal for weight loss and dieting as it is packed with nutrient-dense ingredients that help to keep you feeling full and energised. Here's how to make a smoothie bowl with banana, almond milk, and chia seeds for weight loss and dieting:

1. Start by adding 1 banana to a blender.

2. Pour in ½ cup of almond milk, and blend until smooth.

3. Add 2 tablespoons of chia seeds and blend until combined.

4. Pour the smoothie into a bowl, and top with sliced banana, blueberries, and chia seeds.

5. Enjoy your smoothie bowl for breakfast or as a snack.

This smoothie bowl is high in fibre, protein, and healthy fats, all of which are important for weight loss and dieting. This smoothie bowl is quick to make and can be

customised to your tastes and diet. Enjoy your smoothie bowl and start your day off right!
Preparation time: 10 minutes

Snack
A handful of nuts.

A handful of nuts is a great snack for weight loss and dieting. Not only are they full of healthy fats and protein, but they also provide essential vitamins and minerals. Here's how to make a handful of nuts for weight loss and dieting:

1. Choose your nuts. There are many different types of nuts to choose from, such as almonds, walnuts, cashews, and pistachios. Choose whichever type you prefer or mix and match.

2. Measure out a handful of nuts. A single serving of nuts is typically one ounce or about two tablespoons. This is roughly equivalent to one handful.

3. Roast the nuts. Roasting your nuts can make them more flavorful and crunchy. Preheat your oven to 350°F and spread a single layer of nuts on a baking sheet lined with parchment paper. Bake for 10-15 minutes, stirring once or twice, until golden and fragrant.

4. Add some flavour. Add a pinch of salt or a sprinkle of your favourite spices such as cinnamon, nutmeg, or allspice.

5. Enjoy your healthy snack. Eat your roasted nuts as a snack or sprinkle them over your favourite salads or yoghurt. They make a great addition to any meal!

Making a handful of nuts is an easy and healthy way to add a bit of crunch to your diet. Eating nuts regularly is linked to many health benefits, such as reducing the risk of heart disease and promoting weight loss. So, snack on a handful of nuts and enjoy the health benefits!
Preparation time: 5 minutes

Lunch
Turkey wrap with tomatoes, lettuce, and hummus.

Making a healthy turkey wrap with tomatoes, lettuce, and hummus is a great way to promote weight loss and dieting. to get started:

- 4-6 ounces of sliced turkey
- 1 whole wheat tortilla
- Half a cup of lettuce leaves, shredded
- Half a cup of chopped tomatoes
- 2 tablespoons of hummus

To begin, preheat your oven to 375 degrees. Place the turkey slices onto a baking sheet and bake for 15 minutes.

Meanwhile, lay the tortilla flat on a plate or cutting board. Spread the hummus in an even layer over the entire surface of the wrap.

Next, add the lettuce and tomatoes to the wrap. You can either add them in a single layer or layer them over the hummus.

Once the turkey is done baking, add it to the wrap and roll it up tightly. Place the wrap on a plate and cut it into pieces.

Enjoy your healthy turkey wrap with tomatoes, lettuce, and hummus! This wrap is a great way to promote weight loss and dieting, as it is low in calories and high in protein and fibre.
Preparation time: 10 minutes

Snack
Celery sticks with almond butter.

Making celery sticks with almond butter is a great way to enjoy a nutritious and delicious snack while on a weight loss or dieting plan. Here's how to make them:

1. Start by washing the celery and cutting it into sticks.

2. Spread the almond butter evenly on the celery sticks.

3. Sprinkle with a pinch of salt and pepper, if desired.

4. Enjoy your healthy snack!

Eating celery sticks with almond butter is a great way to get in some extra nutrients while keeping your calorie intake low. Celery is high in dietary fibre and low in calories, while almond butter is a good source of healthy fats and protein. In addition, the combination of these two ingredients provides a great balance of macronutrients and can help you feel fuller for longer. Enjoy this snack as part of your weight loss or dieting plan for a healthy and delicious treat.
Preparation time: 5 minutes

Dinner

Baked sweet potato with grilled shrimp and sautéed vegetables.

Making a delicious and nutritious meal out of Baked Sweet Potato with Grilled Shrimp and Sautéed Vegetables is a great way to help with weight loss and dieting. This meal is low in calories but packed with flavour and nutrition!

First, start by baking the sweet potatoes. Preheat the oven to 375 degrees Fahrenheit and pierce the skin of the potatoes several times with a fork. Place the potatoes on a baking sheet and bake for approximately one hour or until they are tender and can be easily pierced with a fork.

Meanwhile, prepare the remaining ingredients. Peel and devein the shrimp and season with salt, pepper, and garlic powder. Heat a non-stick skillet over medium-high heat and add a tablespoon of olive oil. Once the oil is hot, add the seasoned shrimp and cook for about three minutes, flipping once, until the shrimp are cooked through. Remove the shrimp from the skillet and set aside.

Breakfast

Avocado toast with poached eggs.

Avocado toast with poached eggs is a delicious and healthy breakfast option that is great for anyone looking to follow a healthy diet. To make this delicious breakfast, you will need:

two slices of whole wheat or multigrain bread
1/2 an avocado
2 eggs
Salt and pepper to taste
1 tablespoon of olive oil

Start by bringing the olive oil to medium-high heat in a skillet. The eggs should be cracked into the skillet once the oil is heated. The eggs should be cooked for around five minutes, or until the whites are fully cooked but the yolks are still a little runny, on low heat. From the skillet, take out the eggs, and place them aside.

Next, toast the slices of bread in the toaster until lightly browned. Once the toast is done, spread the avocado over the toast and season with salt and pepper. Place the poached eggs on top of the toast and sprinkle a bit more salt and pepper over the top.

Your avocado toast with poached eggs is now ready to serve. This healthy breakfast is full of protein, healthy fats, and vitamins, making it a great option for anyone looking to lose weight or follow a healthy diet. Enjoy!
Preparation time: 10 minutes

Apple slices with peanut butter.

Making apple slices with peanut butter is a great way to get some extra nutrition into your diet while still maintaining a healthy weight. Here's how to do it:

1. Begin by washing and drying one apple.

2. Cut the apple into slices, discarding the core.

3. Spread a thin layer of natural peanut butter onto each slice.

4. Place the slices onto a plate.

5. Sprinkle a pinch of cinnamon onto each slice.

6. Enjoy!

These apple slices with peanut butter make for a great snack or light meal that is perfect for weight loss and dieting. Natural peanut butter is a great source of healthy fats and protein, while the apple provides a good source of dietary fibre. The cinnamon adds a nice flavour and can help boost your metabolism.
Preparation time: 5 minutes

Lunch
Grilled chicken with quinoa and roasted vegetables.

Ingredients:

-1 lb boneless, skinless chicken breasts
-1 cup quinoa
-1 red bell pepper, cut into strips
-1 yellow bell pepper, cut into strips
-1 zucchini, cut into slices
-1 yellow squash, cut into slices
-1 red onion, cut into wedges
-2 tablespoons olive oil
-1 teaspoon garlic powder
-1 teaspoon dried oregano
-Salt and pepper, to taste
-Fresh parsley, for garnish

Instructions:

1. Preheat your grill to medium-high heat.

2. Heat 2 cups of water to a rolling boil in a medium saucepan. Cook for 15 minutes with the lid on after adding the quinoa and lowering the heat.

3. Combine the bell peppers, yellow squash, zucchini, and red onion in a big bowl. Add the olive oil and season with salt, pepper, oregano, garlic powder, and olive oil. Mix by tossing.

4. After adding the vegetables to the grill, cook them for 4-5 minutes, or until they are tender and just beginning

to char. Cook for an additional 4-5 minutes after flipping the vegetables.

5. Place the chicken on the grill and cook for 8-10 minutes, flipping halfway through.

6. To serve, divide the quinoa onto four plates. Top with the grilled vegetables and chicken. Garnish with fresh parsley, if desired. Enjoy!

Note: To make this dish extra healthy, use skinless, boneless chicken breasts and use olive oil instead of butter.

Preparation time: 15 minutes

Yoghurt with berries.

Ingredients:

-1 cup plain Greek yoghourt
-1 cup frozen mixed berries
-1 tablespoon honey
-1 teaspoon chia seeds
-½ teaspoon ground cinnamon

Instructions:

1. In a medium bowl, combine the Greek yoghurt, frozen mixed berries, honey, chia seeds, and ground cinnamon.

2. Stir until everything is evenly mixed.

3. Place the mixture in a container and store it in the refrigerator until ready to serve.

4. When ready to serve, scoop the yoghurt mixture into a bowl.

Preparation time: 5 minutes

Dinner

Baked salmon with sweet potato and steamed broccoli.

Making a healthy, balanced meal with baked salmon, sweet potato, and steamed broccoli is a great option for weight loss and dieting. All of these ingredients are high in essential vitamins and minerals, as well as being naturally low in fat and calories.

Start by turning on your oven to 350 degrees Fahrenheit to prepare this dish. The sweet potato should be scrubbed and then sliced into cubes. Olive oil should be lightly drizzled over the cubes before placing them on a baking pan covered with parchment paper. Bake the sweet potato for 25 to 30 minutes, or until it's fully done.

Prepare the salmon in the meanwhile. On a baking sheet covered with parchment, spread a fillet of salmon and season with salt and pepper. Salmon should be baked for 15 to 20 minutes, or until a fork can easily pierce it.

Start by turning on your oven to 350 degrees Fahrenheit to prepare this dish. The sweet potato should be scrubbed and then sliced into cubes. Olive oil should be lightly drizzled over the cubes before placing them on a baking pan covered with parchment paper. Bake the sweet potato for 25 to 30 minutes, or until it's fully done.

Prepare the salmon in the meanwhile. On a baking sheet covered with parchment, spread a fillet of salmon and season with salt and pepper. Salmon should be baked for 15 to 20 minutes, or until a fork can easily pierce it.

While the salmon and sweet potato are baked, prepare the steamed broccoli. Wash the broccoli and cut it into florets. Place the broccoli florets in a steaming basket over a pot of boiling water, and steam for 5-7 minutes.

Once everything is cooked, it's time to assemble the dish. Divide the sweet potato, salmon, and steamed broccoli onto individual plates. Serve with a lemon wedge for added flavour.

Preparation time: 20 minutes

Day 10

Breakfast
Avocado toast with poached eggs.

Avocado toast with poached eggs is a delicious and healthy breakfast option that is great for anyone looking to lose weight or follow a healthy diet. To make this delicious breakfast, you will need:

2 pieces of multigrain or whole wheat toast and 12 an avocado
-2 eggs
-1 tablespoon of olive oil, with salt & pepper to taste

Start by bringing the olive oil to medium-high heat in a skillet. The eggs should be cracked into the skillet once the oil is heated. The eggs should be cooked for around five minutes, or until the whites are fully cooked but the yolks are still a little runny, on low heat. From the skillet, take out the eggs, and place them aside.

Next, toast the slices of bread in the toaster until lightly browned. Once the toast is done, spread the avocado over the toast and season with salt and pepper. Place the poached eggs on top of the toast and sprinkle a bit more salt and pepper over the top.

Your avocado toast with poached eggs is now ready to serve. This healthy breakfast is full of protein, healthy fats, and vitamins, making it a great option for anyone looking to lose weight or follow a healthy diet. Enjoy! Preparation time: 10 minutes

Snack
Apple slices with peanut butter.

Making apple slices with peanut butter is a great way to get some extra nutrition into your diet while still maintaining a healthy weight. Here's how to do it:

1. Begin by washing and drying one apple.

2. Cut the apple into slices, discarding the core.

3. Spread a thin layer of natural peanut butter onto each slice.

4. Place the slices onto a plate.

5. Sprinkle a pinch of cinnamon onto each slice.

6. Enjoy!

These apple slices with peanut butter make for a great snack or light meal that is perfect for weight loss and dieting. Natural peanut butter is a great source of healthy fats and protein, while the apple provides a good source of dietary fibre. The cinnamon adds a nice flavour and can help boost your metabolism. Enjoy!

Preparation time: 5 minutes

Grilled chicken with quinoa and roasted vegetables.

Ingredients:

-1 lb boneless, skinless chicken breasts
-1 cup quinoa
-1 red bell pepper, cut into strips
-1 yellow bell pepper, cut into strips
-1 zucchini, cut into slices
-1 yellow squash, cut into slices
-1 red onion, cut into wedges
-2 tablespoons olive oil
-1 teaspoon garlic powder
-1 teaspoon dried oregano
-Salt and pepper, to taste
-Fresh parsley, for garnish

Instructions:

1. Preheat your grill to medium-high heat.

2. Bring two cups of water to a boil in a medium saucepan. For 15 minutes, cook the quinoa while covering the pan and lowering the heat.

3. Combine the yellow squash, zucchini, bell peppers, and red onion in a sizable bowl. Garlic powder, oregano,

salt, and pepper are added after you drizzle on the olive oil. Stir with a toss.

4. Grill the vegetables for 4–5 minutes, or until they are soft and lightly charred. Cook the vegetables for a further 4-5 minutes after flipping.

5. Place the chicken on the grill and cook for 8-10 minutes, flipping halfway through.

6. To serve, divide the quinoa onto four plates. Top with the grilled vegetables and chicken. Garnish with fresh parsley, if desired. Enjoy!

Note: To make this dish extra healthy, use skinless, boneless chicken breasts and use olive oil instead of butter.

Preparation time: 15 minutes

Snack
Yoghurt with berries.

Ingredients:

-1 cup plain Greek yoghourt
-1 cup frozen mixed berries
-1 tablespoon honey
-1 teaspoon chia seeds
-½ teaspoon ground cinnamon

Instructions:

1. In a medium bowl, combine the Greek yoghurt, frozen mixed berries, honey, chia seeds, and ground cinnamon.

2. Stir until everything is evenly mixed.

3. Place the mixture in a container and store it in the refrigerator until ready to serve.

4. When ready to serve, scoop the yoghurt mixture into a bowl.

5. Enjoy!

Preparation time: 5 minutes

Dinner

Baked salmon with sweet potato and steamed broccoli.

Making a healthy, balanced meal with baked salmon, sweet potato, and steamed broccoli is a great option for weight loss and dieting. All of these ingredients are high in essential vitamins and minerals, as well as being naturally low in fat and calories.

Start by turning on your oven to 350 degrees Fahrenheit to prepare this dish. The sweet potato should be scrubbed and then sliced into cubes. Olive oil should be lightly drizzled over the cubes before placing them on a baking pan covered with parchment paper. Bake the sweet potato for 25 to 30 minutes, or until it's fully done.

Prepare the salmon in the meanwhile. On a baking sheet covered with parchment, spread a fillet of salmon and season with salt and pepper. Salmon should be baked for 15 to 20 minutes, or until a fork can easily pierce it.

While the salmon and sweet potato are baked, prepare the steamed broccoli. Wash the broccoli and cut it into florets. Place the broccoli florets in a steaming basket over a pot of boiling water, and steam for 5-7 minutes.

Once everything is cooked, it's time to assemble the dish. Divide the sweet potato, salmon, and steamed

broccoli onto individual plates. Serve with a lemon wedge for an added flavour kick. Enjoy!
Preparation time: 20 minutes

Day 11

Breakfast
Oatmeal with fresh fruit and nuts.

Making oatmeal with fresh fruit and nuts is a great way to start your day for weight loss and dieting. Here are the steps to make delicious and nutritious oatmeal:

1. Gather the ingredients: oats, fresh fruit, nuts, milk, honey, butter

2. Measure out the oats (1/2 cup per person) and put them in a saucepan.

3. Add enough milk to cover the oats and turn the heat on to medium.

4. Once the milk is boiling, add the honey and butter.

5. Simmer the oats for 5 minutes, stirring occasionally.

6. Once the oats are cooked, turn off the heat and stir in the fresh fruit and nuts.

7. Add spices for extra flavour (optional).

8. Serve the oatmeal in bowls and enjoy!

This oatmeal recipe is delicious, nutritious, and perfect for weight loss and dieting. The combination of oats, fresh fruit, nuts, and honey will give you the energy you need to start your day, and the healthy fats and protein will keep you full and energised until lunchtime. Enjoy! Preparation time: 10 minutes

Snack
Celery sticks with hummus.

Making celery sticks with hummus is a great way to enjoy a healthy snack while also aiding in weight loss and dieting. To make this delicious and nutritious snack, you will need:

1. Celery stalks - 1-2 stalks per person

2. Hummus - 1-2 tablespoons per person

3. Optional: Sea salt, freshly ground pepper, paprika, and/or garlic powder

Instructions:

1. Wash and cut the celery stalks into 3-4 inch pieces.

2. Place the celery pieces on a plate.

3. In a small bowl, mix the hummus with a fork or whisk until smooth.

4. Add the hummus to the celery pieces, using a spoon to spread it evenly.

5. Sprinkle with the optional sea salt, freshly ground pepper, paprika, and/or garlic powder.

6. Enjoy your healthy snack!

Eating celery sticks with hummus as a snack or light meal is a great way to enjoy a nutritious and filling snack that can help you reach your weight loss and dieting goals. Enjoy!
Preparation time: 5 minutes

Lunch
Lentil soup with a side of whole wheat toast.

Making Lentil Soup with a side of whole wheat toast for weight loss and dieting is a great way to enjoy a delicious and healthy meal.

Get the following ingredients first before you begin:

- 1 tablespoon olive oil
- 1 small onion, finely chopped
- 2 cloves garlic, minced
- 1 cup of washed and drained dried lentils
- 4 cups vegetable broth
- 2 cups diced tomatoes
- 1 teaspoon dried oregano
- 1 teaspoon dried thyme
- 1/2 teaspoon ground cumin
- Salt and pepper to taste
- Whole wheat toast

Now let's get started!

1. In a big pot, heat the olive oil on medium-high.

2. Add the onion and garlic and sauté until the onion is softened for about 5 minutes.

3. Add the lentils, broth, tomatoes, oregano, thyme, and cumin.

4. Bring the mixture to a boil, then reduce the heat and simmer for about 30 minutes, or until the lentils are tender.

5. Add salt and pepper to taste and turn the heat off.

6. Serve with a side of whole wheat toast.

Enjoy your delicious and healthy Lentil Soup with a side of whole wheat toast!
 Preparation time: 15 minutes

Snack
A handful of nuts.

A handful of nuts is a great snack for weight loss and dieting. Not only are they full of healthy fats and protein, but they also provide essential vitamins and minerals. Here's how to make a handful of nuts for weight loss and dieting:

1. Choose your nuts. There are many different types of nuts to choose from, such as almonds, walnuts, cashews, and pistachios. Choose whichever type you prefer or mix and match.

2. Measure out a handful of nuts. A single serving of nuts is typically one ounce or about two tablespoons. This is roughly equivalent to one handful.

3. Roast the nuts. Roasting your nuts can make them more flavorful and crunchy. Preheat your oven to 350°F and spread a single layer of nuts on a baking sheet lined with parchment paper. Bake for 10-15 minutes, stirring once or twice, until golden and fragrant.

4. Add some flavour. Add a pinch of salt or a sprinkle of your favourite spices such as cinnamon, nutmeg, or allspice.

5. Enjoy your healthy snack. Eat your roasted nuts as a snack or sprinkle them over your favourite salads or yoghurt. They are a good complement to any meal!

Making a handful of nuts is an easy and healthy way to add a bit of crunch to your diet. Eating nuts regularly is linked to many health benefits, such as reducing the risk of heart disease and promoting weight loss. So, snack on a handful of nuts and enjoy the health benefits!

Preparation time: 5 minutes

Dinner
Baked cod with roasted Brussels sprouts and lemon.

Ingredients:

- - 4 fillets of cod (about 6 ounces each)
- 2 tablespoons extra-virgin olive oil
- 2 teaspoons fresh thyme, chopped
- freshly ground black pepper and Kosher salt
- 2 tablespoons capers, drained
- 2 garlic cloves, minced
- 2 tablespoons freshly squeezed lemon juice
- 2 tablespoons dry white wine
- 1-2 cups halved and trimmed Brussels sprouts
- 2 tablespoons olive oil

Instructions:

1. Set the oven's temperature to 400 F.

2. Sprinkle the cod fillets with thyme, salt, and pepper.

3. In a small bowl, mix the capers, garlic, lemon juice, and white wine.

4. Place the cod fillets in a baking dish and pour the caper mixture over them.

5. Place the Brussels sprouts in a separate baking dish and drizzle with olive oil.

6. Place both dishes in the preheated oven and bake for 15 minutes.

7. Remove the cod from the oven and let it rest for 5 minutes.

8. Serve the cod with Brussels sprouts and a lemon wedge.

 Preparation time: 20 minutes

Day 12

Breakfast
Scrambled egg whites with spinach and mushrooms.

Scrambled egg whites with spinach and mushrooms are a great way to get protein, fibre, and vitamins while on a weight loss and dieting plan. Here's how to make them:

1. A nonstick pan should first be heated over low heat.

2. Once heated, add 2 tablespoons of olive oil or butter.

3. Then add 1 cup of sliced mushrooms, 1 cup of chopped spinach, and 1/4 teaspoon of salt.

4. Saute the vegetables for 2-3 minutes until softened.

5. Then add 1/4 cup of egg whites and scramble until cooked through.

6. Serve hot with a side of your favourite toast.

These scrambled egg whites with spinach and mushrooms are a delicious and nutritious way to start your day. Enjoy!

Preparation time: 10 minutes

Apple slices with peanut butter.

Making apple slices with peanut butter is a great snack for those trying to lose weight or maintain a healthy diet. Here are the steps to prepare this tasty snack:

1. Start by washing your apple thoroughly. Cut it into thin, 1/4-inch-thick wedges.

2. On each slice, apply a thin layer of peanut butter.

3. Place the slices on a plate and refrigerate until ready to eat.

4. Enjoy your healthy snack!

This snack is a great way to get some protein and healthy fats without going overboard in either category. The peanut butter also provides some sweetness, while the apple brings in some important vitamins and minerals. Enjoy this snack as part of a balanced diet for weight loss or maintenance.

Preparation time: 5 minutes

Greek salad with grilled chicken, feta cheese, and olives.

Greek salad with grilled chicken, feta cheese, and olives is a delicious and healthy meal that can be enjoyed as part of a weight loss and diet plan. The combination of fresh greens, lean protein, and healthy fats make this salad a great choice for anyone looking to lose weight and maintain a healthy lifestyle. Here's how to make it:

1. Start by preparing the ingredients. Rinse and then chop 1 head of romaine lettuce and 1 large cucumber. Slice 1 red onion and 1 bell pepper into thin strips. Cut 1/2 cup of pitted kalamata olives in half.

2. Grill 8 ounces of boneless, skinless chicken breasts. Once cooked through, let cool before slicing into thin strips.

3. In a large bowl, combine the prepared lettuce, cucumber, onion, bell pepper, and olives.

4. Add the chicken strips and a generous sprinkle of feta cheese.

5. Drizzle with a light vinaigrette dressing and mix everything.

6. Enjoy your Greek salad with grilled chicken, feta cheese, and olives. It's a great way to get a healthy

dose of vegetables and protein while still eating a delicious meal.
Preparation time: 15 minutes

Snack
Celery sticks with almond butter.

Making celery sticks with almond butter is an easy way to add a nutritious and delicious snack to your weight loss and dieting plan. Here's how to make it:

1. Start by washing and cutting up 2-4 celery stalks into 2-4 inch pieces.

2. Spread a tablespoon of almond butter onto each piece of celery.

3. Sprinkle with your favourite healthy toppings such as chia seeds, hemp hearts, or chopped nuts.

4. Enjoy as a healthy snack or as an accompaniment to a meal.

Eating celery sticks with almond butter is a great way to get in some extra fibre, protein, and healthy fats. This snack is low in calories and is great for weight loss and dieting. Plus, it's quick and easy to make, making it a great option for busy days. Enjoy!
Preparation time: 5 minutes

Baked sweet potato with grilled shrimp and steamed vegetables.

Ingredients:

-1 large sweet potato
-1/2 pound of large shrimp
-1/2 cup of vegetable broth
-1/2 cup of diced bell peppers
-1/2 cup of diced carrots
-1/2 cup of diced zucchini
-1 tablespoon of olive oil
-Salt and pepper to taste

Instructions:

1. The oven should be preheated to 375 degrees.

2. Wash the sweet potato and prick holes all around it with a fork. Place on a baking sheet and bake for 45 minutes, or until it is soft when you press it.

3. In a medium bowl, mix the shrimp with vegetable broth, bell peppers, carrots, and zucchini.

4. In a big skillet over medium heat, warm the olive oil. Add the shrimp and vegetable mixture and cook for 3-4 minutes, or until the shrimp is cooked through and the vegetables are tender. add salt and pepper to the food. To taste

5. Cut the baked sweet potato in half, and top with the shrimp and vegetables. Serve warm.

This meal is perfect for weight loss and dieting, as it is packed with nutrients and low in calories. The sweet potato is a great source of dietary fibre and complex carbohydrates, while the shrimp and vegetables provide lean protein and vitamins. Enjoy!
Preparation time: 20 minutes

Day 13

Overnight oats with banana and almond butter.
Overnight oats with banana and almond butter make for an incredibly satisfying and nutritious breakfast. They are a great way to start the day, provide plenty of dietary fibre, and can even help with weight loss and dieting. Here's how to make them:

1. Start by combining 1 cup of old-fashioned oats and 1 cup of milk (or your favourite non-dairy milk) in a bowl and stir together.

2. Add 1 banana, mashed, and 2 tablespoons of almond butter. Stir everything together completely.

3. Place the bowl in the refrigerator overnight.

4. In the morning, you will have a delicious, creamy breakfast ready to eat.

For an extra boost of flavour, you can top your oats with your favourite fruits, nuts, or seeds. There are endless possibilities!

Overnight oats with banana and almond butter are a great way to get your day off to a healthy start. They are easy to make, packed with nutrition, and can help with weight loss and dieting. Enjoy!

Preparation time: 10 minutes

Snack

A handful of nuts.

A handful of nuts is a great snack for weight loss and dieting. Not only are they full of healthy fats and protein, but they also provide essential vitamins and minerals. Here's how to make a handful of nuts for weight loss and dieting:

1. Choose your nuts. There are many different types of nuts to choose from, such as almonds, walnuts, cashews, and pistachios. Choose whichever type you prefer or mix and match.

2. Measure out a handful of nuts. A single serving of nuts is typically one ounce or about two tablespoons. This is roughly equivalent to one handful.

3. Roast the nuts. Roasting your nuts can make them more flavorful and crunchy. Preheat your oven to 350°F and spread a single layer of nuts on a baking sheet lined with parchment paper. Bake for 10-15 minutes, stirring once or twice, until golden and fragrant.

4. Add some flavour. Add a pinch of salt or a sprinkle of your favourite spices such as cinnamon, nutmeg, or allspice.

5. Enjoy your healthy snack. Eat your roasted nuts as a snack or sprinkle them over your favourite salads or yoghurt. They are a wonderful meal!

Making a handful of nuts is an easy and healthy way to add a bit of crunch to your diet. Eating nuts regularly is linked to many health benefits, such as reducing the risk of heart disease and promoting weight loss. So, snack on a handful of nuts and enjoy the health benefits!

Preparation time: 5 minutes

Lunch
Kale salad with grilled chicken, tomatoes, and balsamic vinaigrette.

Making a Kale Salad with Grilled Chicken, Tomatoes and Balsamic Vinaigrette is a great way to get your daily recommended intake of vegetables, lean protein, and healthy fats. This salad is perfect for weight loss and dieting since it is low in calories, high in fibre, and packed with nutrients. Here's how to make it:

1. Start by prepping the kale. Rinse off the leaves and discard any thick stems. Then tear the leaves into bite-sized pieces and place them in a large bowl.

2. Next, prepare the grilled chicken.
 Fire up the grill and sprinkle salt and pepper on the chicken.   Grill the chicken until it's cooked through,

about 4-5 minutes per side. Once it's done, let it cool before slicing it into thin strips.

3. Add the grilled chicken to the bowl with the kale. Then, slice some fresh tomatoes and add them to the bowl.

4. Finally, make the balsamic vinaigrette. In a small bowl, whisk together ¼ cup of balsamic vinegar, ½ cup of extra-virgin olive oil, 1 tablespoon of Dijon mustard, 1 teaspoon of honey, 1 minced garlic clove, along with a little salt and pepper.

5. Pour the vinaigrette over the salad and toss it all together. Serve the salad immediately and enjoy!
Preparation time: 15 minutes

Snack

Yoghurt with berries.

Making yoghurt with berries for weight loss and dieting can be an easy and delicious way to improve your health and help you reach your dieting goals.

To get started, you'll need 1 cup of plain Greek yoghurt, 1/2 cup of frozen berries (such as strawberries, blueberries, and raspberries), 1 tablespoon of honey, and 1 teaspoon of vanilla extract.

First, combine the yoghurt, honey, and vanilla extract in a bowl and mix until completely combined.

Next, add the frozen berries and stir until they are evenly distributed throughout the yoghurt.

Once everything is combined, pour the yoghurt mixture into a container and place it in the refrigerator to chill for at least 1 hour.

When ready to eat, scoop out a portion of the yoghurt and top it with your favourite fresh berries. Enjoy!

Yoghurt with berries is an excellent snack for weight loss and dieting because it is high in protein, low in fat, and full of antioxidants and vitamins. The protein helps keep you feeling full longer, while the antioxidants in the berries help to reduce inflammation, promote healthy weight loss, and boost your immune system.

about how to make Yogurt with berries for weight loss and dieting

Making yoghurt with berries for weight loss and dieting can be an easy and delicious way to improve your health and help you reach your dieting goals.

To get started, you'll need 1 cup of plain Greek yoghurt, 1/2 cup of frozen berries (such as strawberries, blueberries, and raspberries), 1 tablespoon of honey, and 1 teaspoon of vanilla extract.

First, combine the yoghurt, honey, and vanilla extract in a bowl and mix until completely combined.

Next, add the frozen berries and stir until they are evenly distributed throughout the yoghurt.

Once everything is combined, pour the yoghurt mixture into a container and place it in the refrigerator to chill for at least 1 hour.

Dinner
Baked salmon with quinoa and roasted Brussels sprouts.

Ingredients

- 4 (4-ounce) salmon fillets
- 1 teaspoon olive oil
- To taste, add salt and freshly ground black pepper.
- 1 cup cooked quinoa
 - two cups of halved and trimmed Brussels sprouts
- 2 tablespoons olive oil
- 2 cloves garlic, minced
- 2 tablespoons freshly squeezed lemon juice
- 2 tablespoons chopped parsley

Instructions

1. Preheat the oven to 400°F. A 9x13 baking dish should be lightly oiled or coated with nonstick spray.

2. Place salmon fillets in the prepared baking dish and season with salt and pepper, to taste. Drizzle with olive oil.

3. Place Brussels sprouts in a separate bowl and toss with olive oil, garlic, lemon juice, and parsley; season with salt and pepper, to taste.

4. Place Brussels sprouts in the baking dish with the salmon.

5. Bake salmon and Brussels sprouts for 15-20 minutes, or until salmon is cooked through.

6. Serve salmon with quinoa and Brussels sprouts. Enjoy!
Preparation time: 20 minutes

Day 14

Breakfast

Smoothie bowl with banana, almond milk, and chia seeds.

Making a smoothie bowl with banana, almond milk, and chia seeds is an easy and nutritious way to start your day. This smoothie bowl is especially beneficial for those looking to lose weight and improve their overall diet.

To make the smoothie bowl, start by adding one banana, one cup of almond milk, and one tablespoon of chia seeds into a blender. The ingredients should be thoroughly blended.

Next, pour the smoothie mixture into a bowl and top with desired toppings. Great options for toppings include granola, nuts, fresh fruit, and shredded coconut.

When you're ready to eat, the smoothie bowl should be chilled and thick. Eating it with a spoon will help you to get the most out of each bite.

Bananas are packed with potassium and provide essential vitamins and minerals. Almond milk is a great source of protein and can help keep you feeling fuller for longer. Chia seeds are high in fibre, which helps to reduce cholesterol levels and reduce the risk of heart disease.

By combining these ingredients into a smoothie bowl, you can get all the benefits of a nutritious breakfast without the added sugar and calories of processed foods. This smoothie bowl is an ideal way to jumpstart your day and begin your weight loss journey
 Preparation time: 10 minutes

Snack
Apple slices with peanut butter.

Apple slices with peanut butter are a great snack option for weight loss and dieting as it is a low-calorie and high-fibre snack.

To start, select an apple that is ripe and has a good texture. Peel the skin off the apple and cut it into even slices. Place the apple slices on a plate and spread a thin layer of peanut butter on each slice. The peanut butter should be very spreadable and not too thick.

Next, sprinkle a few chopped nuts on top of the peanut butter-covered apple slices. This will add some extra flavour and texture to the snack.

Finally, cover the plate with plastic wrap and put it in the refrigerator for about an hour. For the flavours to blend.

When you are ready to eat, take out the plate of apple slices with peanut butter and enjoy. This snack is a

great way to satisfy hunger and will help keep you feeling full for hours. Plus, it is low in calories and high in fibre, making it an ideal snack for weight loss and dieting. Enjoy!
 Preparation time: 5 minutes

Lunch
Turkey wrap with tomatoes, lettuce, and hummus.

Making a turkey wrap with tomatoes, lettuce, and hummus is a great way to enjoy a healthy and delicious meal for weight loss and dieting. Here is how to make it:

1. Start by gathering the ingredients: 2-3 slices of turkey, 2-3 slices of tomato, 1-2 large lettuce leaves, 2-3 tablespoons of hummus, and whole-wheat wrap.

2. Spread the hummus on the wrap.

3. Place the slices of turkey on the wrap.

4. Top with the tomato slices and lettuce leaves.

5. Roll up the wrap, tucking in the sides as you go.

6. Cut the wrap in half diagonally and serve.

This turkey wrap is a great source of protein and healthy fats, and tomatoes, lettuce, and hummus provide a good source of vitamins and minerals. Enjoy this healthy and delicious wrap for weight loss and dieting!

Preparation time: 10 minutes

Snack

Celery sticks with almond butter.

Making celery sticks with almond butter is a great way to enjoy a healthy snack while losing weight. It's low in calories, high in fibre, and packed with essential nutrients. Here's how to make this tasty treat:

1. Start by washing and cutting the celery into 4-inch sticks.

2. Spread a thin layer of almond butter on each celery stick.

3. Sprinkle with your favourite seasonings, such as sea salt, garlic powder, or black pepper.

4. Place the celery sticks on a plate and enjoy!

This snack is a great way to get your daily dose of fibre, healthy fats, and protein while sticking to your diet. The almond butter adds a nutty flavour and creamy texture, while the celery provides a crunchy and refreshing taste. You can also top the celery sticks with other ingredients,

such as raisins, sunflower seeds, or hemp hearts, to add
an extra layer of flavour and nutrition. Enjoy!
Preparation time: 5 minutes

Dinner

Baked cod with steamed cauliflower and lemon.

This healthy, delicious, and easy-to-make dish is the
perfect meal for weight loss and dieting. To make Baked
Cod with Steamed Cauliflower and Lemon, you will
need:

- 6-ounce cod fillet
- 1 head cauliflower, cut into florets
- 2 tablespoons olive oil
- Salt and pepper
- 1 lemon, thinly sliced
- 2 tablespoons chopped fresh parsley

Instructions:

1. Preheat the oven to 425°F.

2. Place the cod fillet in a baking dish. Add salt and
pepper, Add salt and pepper and spray some oil.

3. Bake cod in a preheated oven for 15 minutes, or until
cooked through.

4. Meanwhile, steam cauliflower florets in a steamer
basket or steam them in a pot with a little bit of water.
Steam for 8 minutes, or until tender.

5. Transfer cod to a plate and top with steamed cauliflower. Sprinkle with parsley and serve. Enjoy!
Preparation time: 15 minutes

Day 15

Breakfast:
Avocado toast with poached eggs.

Ingredients:

- 2 slices of whole wheat bread
- 1 ripe avocado
- 1 teaspoon of lemon juice
- Salt and pepper to taste
- 2 eggs
- 2 tablespoons of white vinegar

Instructions:

1. Start by toasting the bread in a toaster or a pan over medium heat.

2. While the bread is toasting, cut the avocado in half, remove the seed and mash the flesh in a small bowl.

3. Add the lemon juice, salt, and pepper and mix until it forms a paste.

4. Once the bread is toasted, spread the avocado paste over each slice.

5. Poach the eggs by bringing a pot of water to a simmer and adding the vinegar.

6. Crack each egg into the simmering water and poach for about 3-4 minutes.

7. Remove the eggs with a slotted spoon and place them on top of the avocado toast.

8. Sprinkle it with additional salt and pepper to taste and enjoy!

For those looking to lose weight and diet, this is a great option as it is low in calories and packed with protein, healthy fats, and vitamins and minerals. The whole wheat bread provides fibre and the eggs supply protein to keep you full and satiated. Plus, the healthy fats from the avocado help to slow down digestion to keep you feeling full for longer. Enjoy!
Preparation time: 10 minutes

Snack
A handful of nuts.

Handfuls of nuts are an excellent snack for weight loss and dieting. They are high in fibre, protein, and healthy fats, all of which help to keep you feeling full and satisfied. Here are some tips for incorporating handfuls of nuts into your weight loss and dieting plan:

1. Choose a variety of nuts. Different types of nuts offer different health benefits, so it's best to mix them up. Whether you prefer almonds, walnuts, cashews,

macadamias, or some other variety, you'll get a variety of vitamins, minerals, and antioxidants from your snack.

2. Opt for raw and unsalted nuts. Roasted and salted varieties may be more flavorful, but they are typically higher in calories and sodium.

3. Keep portion sizes in check. Although nuts are nutrient-dense, they are still calorie-dense. A single handful of nuts can contain anywhere from 150 to 300 calories. Therefore, it's important to be mindful of portion sizes.

4. Incorporate nuts into meals. Handfuls of nuts are not only great snacks but they can also be incorporated into meals. Add a handful of chopped nuts to salads or oatmeal for an extra crunch and added nutrition.

5. Eat nuts with other healthy foods. Eating nuts alone can lead to overeating. To avoid over-snacking, pair them with other healthy foods, such as fruits and vegetables.

By following these tips, you can make handfuls of nuts a part of your weight loss and dieting plan. Not only are they tasty, but they are also an excellent source of vitamins, minerals, and healthy fats.
 Preparation time: 5 minutes

Lunch
Quinoa bowl with grilled chicken, tomatoes, and balsamic vinaigrette.

Making a quinoa bowl with grilled chicken, tomatoes, and balsamic vinaigrette is a great way to enjoy a healthy, balanced meal while still keeping your diet on track. Quinoa is a superfood that is packed with protein, fibre, and other essential vitamins and minerals. Combined with the lean protein of grilled chicken, tomatoes for added vitamin C, and a flavorful balsamic vinaigrette, this meal is sure to keep you on track for weight loss and dieting.

To make this quinoa bowl, start by preparing the quinoa according to the package instructions. Once cooked, fluff the quinoa and transfer it to a large bowl.

While the quinoa is cooking, prepare the grilled chicken. Heat a large skillet over medium-high heat, and then add a tablespoon of olive oil. Add the chicken breasts to the pan and cook for about five minutes on each side, or until the chicken is cooked through.

Next, prepare the tomatoes. Slice two tomatoes into thin slices and place them in a separate bowl.

To make the balsamic vinaigrette, combine one tablespoon of balsamic vinegar, two tablespoons of olive oil, one teaspoon of honey, and a pinch of salt and pepper in a small bowl. Whisk until everything is combined.

Once everything is prepared, add the grilled chicken, tomatoes, and balsamic vinaigrette to the bowl of quinoa. Toss the ingredients together until everything is evenly combined.

Serve the quinoa bowl with grilled chicken, tomatoes, and balsamic vinaigrette immediately. Enjoy!
Preparation time: 15 minutes

Snack
Whole wheat crackers with cottage cheese.

Making whole wheat crackers with cottage cheese is a great way to enjoy a healthy snack while on a weight loss and dieting plan. These crackers are high in protein, low in fat, and have a great crunchy texture that is perfect for satisfying a snack craving.

To make whole wheat crackers with cottage cheese, you will need 1 cup of whole wheat flour, 1 cup of cottage cheese, 1 teaspoon of baking powder, and 1/2 teaspoon of salt.

Start by preheating your oven to 375 degrees Fahrenheit. In a large bowl, mix the flour, cottage cheese, baking powder, and salt until combined. You may need to use your hands to mix the dough if it becomes too thick.

Next, turn the dough onto a lightly floured surface and roll it out until it is about 1/4 inch thick. Cut the dough into small cracker-sized pieces and place them on a greased baking sheet.

Bake for about 15 minutes or until the crackers are golden brown. Allow the crackers to cool before serving.

These whole wheat crackers with cottage cheese make a great snack for weight loss and dieting. Not only are they low in fat, but they also provide a great source of protein and fibre. Enjoy!

Preparation time: 5 minutes

Baked sweet potato with grilled shrimp and sautéed vegetables.

Ingredients

- 2 sweet potatoes, scrubbed and cut into cubes
- 1/2 pound medium shrimp, peeled and deveined
- 2 tablespoons olive oil
- 1 red bell pepper, diced
- 1 yellow bell pepper, diced
- 1/2 red onion, diced
- 2 cloves garlic, minced
- 1 teaspoon chilli powder
- 1 teaspoon smoked paprika
- 1/2 teaspoon ground cumin
- 1/4 teaspoon sea salt
- 1/4 teaspoon ground black pepper

Instructions

1. Preheat the oven to 400°F. Place sweet potato cubes on a baking sheet and lightly coat with cooking spray or olive oil. Bake for 25 minutes or until tender.

2. Heat olive oil in a large skillet over medium-high heat. Add the shrimp and cook for 3 minutes.

3. Add the bell peppers, onion, garlic, chilli powder, smoked paprika, cumin, salt, and pepper. Cook, stirring

occasionally, for an additional 5 minutes or until vegetables are tender.

4. Serve the grilled shrimp and vegetables on top of the sweet potatoes. Enjoy!
Preparation time: 20 minutes

Day 16

Breakfast: Avocado toast with poached eggs.

Ingredients:

- 2 slices of whole wheat bread
- 1 ripe avocado
- 1 teaspoon of lemon juice
- Salt and pepper to taste
- 2 eggs
- 2 tablespoons of white vinegar

Instructions:

1. Start by toasting the bread in a toaster or a pan over medium heat.

2. While the bread is toasting, cut the avocado in half, remove the seed and mash the flesh in a small bowl.

3. Add the lemon juice, salt, and pepper and mix until it forms a paste.

4. Once the bread is toasted, spread the avocado paste over each slice.

5. Poach the eggs by bringing a pot of water to a simmer and adding the vinegar.

6. Crack each egg into the simmering water and poach for about 3-4 minutes.

7. Remove the eggs with a slotted spoon and place them on top of the avocado toast.

8. Sprinkle it with additional salt and pepper to taste and enjoy!

For those looking to lose weight and diet, this is a great option as it is low in calories and packed with protein, healthy fats, and vitamins and minerals. The whole wheat bread provides fibre and the eggs supply protein to keep you full and satiated. Plus, the healthy fats from the avocado help to slow down digestion to keep you feeling full for longer. Enjoy!
Preparation time: 10 minutes

Snack
A handful of nuts.

Handfuls of nuts are an excellent snack for weight loss and dieting. They are high in fibre, protein, and healthy fats, all of which help to keep you feeling full and satisfied. Here are some tips for incorporating handfuls of nuts into your weight loss and dieting plan:

1. Choose a variety of nuts. Different types of nuts offer different health benefits, so it's best to mix them up. Whether you prefer almonds, walnuts, cashews, macadamias, or some other variety, you'll get a variety of vitamins, minerals, and antioxidants from your snack.

2. Opt for raw and unsalted nuts. Roasted and salted varieties may be more flavorful, but they are typically higher in calories and sodium.

3. Keep portion sizes in check. Although nuts are nutrient-dense, they are still calorie-dense. A single handful of nuts can contain anywhere from 150 to 300 calories. Therefore, it's important to be mindful of portion sizes.

4. Incorporate nuts into meals. Handfuls of nuts are not only great snacks but they can also be incorporated into meals. Add a handful of chopped nuts to salads or oatmeal for an extra crunch and added nutrition.

5. Eat nuts with other healthy foods. Eating nuts alone can lead to overeating. To avoid over-snacking, pair them with other healthy foods, such as fruits and vegetables.

By following these tips, you can make handfuls of nuts a part of your weight loss and dieting plan. Not only are they tasty, but they are also an excellent source of vitamins, minerals, and healthy fats.

Preparation time: 5 minutes

Lunch
Quinoa bowl with grilled chicken, tomatoes, and balsamic vinaigrette.

Making a quinoa bowl with grilled chicken, tomatoes, and balsamic vinaigrette is a great way to enjoy a healthy, balanced meal while still keeping your diet on track. Quinoa is a superfood that is packed with protein, fibre, and other essential vitamins and minerals. Combined with the lean protein of grilled chicken, tomatoes for added vitamin C, and a flavorful balsamic vinaigrette, this meal is sure to keep you on track for weight loss and dieting.

To make this quinoa bowl, start by preparing the quinoa according to the package instructions. Once cooked, fluff the quinoa and transfer it to a large bowl.

While the quinoa is cooking, prepare the grilled chicken. Heat a large skillet over medium-high heat, and then add a tablespoon of olive oil. Add the chicken breasts to the pan and cook for about five minutes on each side, or until the chicken is cooked through.

Next, prepare the tomatoes. Slice two tomatoes into thin slices and place them in a separate bowl.

To make the balsamic vinaigrette, combine one tablespoon of balsamic vinegar, two tablespoons of olive oil, one teaspoon of honey, and a pinch of salt and pepper in a small bowl. Whisk until everything is combined.

Once everything is prepared, add the grilled chicken, tomatoes, and balsamic vinaigrette to the bowl of quinoa. Toss the ingredients together until they are completely mixed.

Serve the quinoa bowl with grilled chicken, tomatoes, and balsamic vinaigrette immediately. Enjoy!
Preparation time: 15 minutes

Whole wheat crackers with cottage cheese.

Making whole wheat crackers with cottage cheese is a great way to enjoy a healthy snack while on a weight loss and dieting plan. These crackers are high in protein, low in fat, and have a great crunchy texture that is perfect for satisfying a snack craving.

To make whole wheat crackers with cottage cheese, you will need 1 cup of whole wheat flour, 1 cup of cottage cheese, 1 teaspoon of baking powder, and 1/2 teaspoon of salt.

Preheat your oven to 375 degrees Fahrenheit. In a large bowl, mix the flour, cottage cheese, baking powder, and salt until combined. You may need to use your hands to mix the dough if it becomes too thick.

Next, turn the dough onto a lightly floured surface and roll it out until it is about 1/4 inch thick. Cut the dough into small cracker-sized pieces and place them on a greased baking sheet.

Bake for about 15 minutes or until the crackers are golden brown. Allow cool before serving.

These whole wheat crackers with cottage cheese make a great snack for weight loss and dieting. Not only are they low in fat, but they also provide a great source of protein and fibre. Enjoy!

Preparation time: 5 minutes

Dinner
Baked salmon with quinoa and roasted Brussels sprouts.

Baked Salmon with Quinoa and Roasted Brussels Sprouts is a great meal for those looking to lose weight and eat a healthy diet. Here's how to make it:

Ingredients:

- 4 salmon fillets
- 2 cups cooked quinoa
- 2 cups Brussels sprouts, halved
- 2 tablespoons olive oil
- Salt and pepper to taste
- 1 lemon, cut into wedges

Instructions:

1. Preheat the oven to 375°F.

2. Salmon fillets should be put on a baking pan. Sprinkle it with salt, pepper, and olive oil.

3. In a separate bowl, combine the quinoa, Brussels sprouts, and the remaining olive oil. Season with salt and pepper.

4. Place the quinoa and Brussels sprouts mixture around the salmon fillets on the baking sheet.

5. Bake in the oven for 20-25 minutes, or until the salmon is cooked through and the Brussels sprouts are lightly browned.

6. Serve with lemon wedges. Enjoy!
 Preparation time: 20 minutes

Day 17

Breakfast
Oatmeal with fresh fruit and nuts.

Ingredients:

-1/2 cup of old-fashioned oats
-1 cup of milk (or nut milk)
-1 teaspoon of honey
-1/2 cup of fresh fruit (berries, pears, apples, etc.)
-2 tablespoons of chopped nuts (almonds, walnuts, pecans, etc.)

Instructions:

1. In a medium saucepan, bring the milk to a gentle simmer.

2. Add the oats and stir to combine. Simmer for 4-5 minutes, stirring occasionally.

3. Add the honey and stir to combine. Simmer for another minute.

4. Remove from heat and transfer the oatmeal to a bowl.

5. Top with fresh fruit and nuts. Enjoy!

Tips for Weight Loss and Dieting:

-Choose low-fat milk or almond milk to reduce the calories.

-Swap out the honey for a natural sweetener, like stevia, for added health benefits.

-Add a tablespoon of chia seeds for an added protein boost.

-Try adding a few tablespoons of plain Greek yoghurt for added creaminess.

-spray cinnamon for added flavour.

 Preparation time: 10 minutes

Snack

A handful of nuts.

Making a Handful of Nuts for weight loss and dieting is a simple and healthy snack that can be enjoyed at any time of day. Here is how to make it:

1. Choose your favourite type of nut. A handful of nuts should contain 1-2 ounces of nuts. Popular choices include almonds, walnuts, cashews, and pistachios.

2. Measure out a single handful of your chosen nut. A single handful should contain 1-2 ounces of nuts.

3. Toast the nuts, if desired. Toasting the nuts will help bring out their flavour and make them crunchier.

4. Sprinkle some sea salt over the nuts, if desired.

5. Place the nuts in a small bowl or container.

6. Enjoy your Handful of Nuts!

Handfuls of nuts are a tasty and nutritious snack that can help keep you full and provide energy. With the right combination of nuts, they can be part of a healthy diet and weight loss plan.
Preparation time: 5 minutes

Lunch
Lentil soup with a side of whole wheat toast.

To make Lentil Soup with a side of whole wheat toast, you will need the following ingredients:

-1 cup dried lentils
-2 cups vegetable or chicken broth
-1 medium onion, diced
-1 carrot, diced
-1 celery stalk, diced
-1 garlic clove, minced
-1 teaspoon ground cumin
-1 teaspoon dried oregano
-1 bay leaf
-Salt and pepper to taste
-2 tablespoons olive oil
-Whole wheat bread for toasting

Instructions:

1. Begin by soaking the lentils in a bowl of cold water for at least 1 hour.

2. Olive oil should be heated in a sizable pot over medium heat. About 5 minutes after adding them, the onion, carrot, celery, and garlic should be tender.

3. Add the cumin, oregano, bay leaf, and a pinch of salt and pepper to the pot. Mix and cook for another minute.

4. Add the soaked lentils and broth to the pot and bring to a boil. Reduce the heat to low and simmer for about 20 minutes or until the lentils are tender.

5. Toast the whole wheat bread.

6. Serve the soup with a side of whole wheat toast. Enjoy!

 Preparation time: 15 minutes

Celery sticks with almond butter.

Making celery sticks with almond butter is an easy and healthy snack option that can be used to help with weight loss and dieting. Here are the steps to make this tasty snack:

1. Start by washing and drying your celery stalks. Before usage, make sure they are clean.

2. Cut the celery into thin slices and arrange them on a plate.

3. Take a spoonful of almond butter and spread it onto each slice of celery.

4. Add a sprinkle of cinnamon or other herbs, if desired.

5. Serve the celery sticks with almond butter as a snack or side dish.

This snack is low in calories but packed with protein and healthy fats from the almond butter. Celery is also a good source of fibre and other vitamins and minerals that can help support weight loss. Enjoy your celery sticks with almond butter as a healthy snack or side dish!
Preparation time: 5 minutes

Dinner

Baked cod with roasted Brussels sprouts and lemon.

Ingredients:

- 4 Cod fillets
- 2 cups halved and trimmed Brussels sprouts
- 2 tablespoons olive oil
- Juice of 1 lemon
- Salt and pepper to taste

Instructions:

1. Preheat the oven to 375°F.

2. Place cod fillets in a baking dish. Drizzle with olive oil and lemon juice, and season with salt and pepper.

3. Place Brussels sprouts in a separate baking dish. Add salt and pepper, then drizzle with olive oil and lemon juice.

4. Bake both dishes in the preheated oven for 25 minutes.

5. Serve the cod and Brussels sprouts together with extra lemon wedges, if desired. Enjoy!
Preparation time: 20 minutes

Day 18

Breakfast
Avocado toast with poached eggs.

Ingredients:
- 4 (6-ounce) cod fillets
- 1 pound Brussels sprouts, trimmed and halved
- 1 lemon, thinly sliced
- 2 tablespoons olive oil
- Salt and freshly ground black pepper
- -2 tablespoons freshly sliced parsley or chives

Instructions:
1. Preheat the oven to 400 degrees F.
2. Cod fillets should be placed on a baking pan covered with parchment paper.
3. Place Brussels sprouts around the cod fillets, and top with lemon slices.
4. Drizzle olive oil over the cod and Brussels sprouts, and season with salt and pepper.
5. Roast in a preheated oven for 20 minutes.
6. Sprinkle with fresh parsley or chives, and serve.

To make this a healthy meal for weight loss and dieting, you can adjust the ingredients and preparation methods. Choose a lower-fat cod, such as Alaskan Pollock or Atlantic cod. Switch out the olive oil for a lower-calorie cooking spray. Instead of roasting the Brussels sprouts, you can steam them to reduce the amount of fat and calories in the dish. If desired, you can also omit the lemon slices to further reduce the calorie content.

Preparation time: 10 minutes

Snack
Apple slices with peanut butter.

1. The first step is to preheat your oven to 350 degrees.

2. Slice your apples into thin slices and spread them on a baking sheet.

3. Spread a thin layer of peanut butter on each slice.

4. Bake in the preheated oven for 10-15 minutes until the apples are softened and lightly browned.

5. Let cool for a few minutes before serving.

These tasty apple slices with peanut butter make a great snack or dessert option for weight loss and dieting. Apples are a good source of vitamins and minerals, and peanut butter adds healthy fats and protein. Eating a few of these slices can help keep you full and satisfied while providing important nutrients that help support your weight loss goals.

Preparation time: 5 minutes

Lunch

Greek salad with grilled chicken, feta cheese, and olives.

Greek salad with grilled chicken, feta cheese, and olives is a quick and easy way to make a delicious and healthy meal. Here is how to make it:

1. SMoking starts by preparing the ingredients.Salt and pepper the chicken after cutting it into cubes. Grill the chicken until cooked through. Cut the cucumbers and tomatoes into cubes, and slice the olives.

2. In a large bowl, mix the cucumbers, tomatoes, olives, feta cheese, and grilled chicken.

3. To make the dressing, mix olive oil, red wine vinegar, garlic, oregano, and a pinch of salt and pepper. Drizzle the dressing over the salad and mix it all.

4. Serve the salad in individual bowls and add a sprinkle of fresh parsley on top. Enjoy!

This Greek salad is a perfect meal for weight loss and dieting. The grilled chicken is low in fat and calories, the vegetables are full of fibre and vitamins, and the olives and feta cheese are full of healthy fats. Enjoy this delicious and healthy meal!
Preparation time: 15 minutes

Yoghurt with berries.

Making yoghurt with berries is a great way to start your day with a healthy and nutritious breakfast. It's low in calories, full of beneficial bacteria, and a great source of fibre and protein. Plus, it's easy to customise with your favourite fruits and toppings. Here's how to make yoghurt with berries for weight loss and dieting.

1. Start by gathering your ingredients. You'll need yoghurt (plain, Greek, or non-dairy), fresh or frozen berries, honey (optional), and any other toppings you'd like.

2. Place the yoghurt in a bowl and add your favourite berries. Mash the berries with a fork to break them up a bit and make them easier to mix.

3. Drizzle some honey over the yoghurt and berries for a hint of sweetness.

4. Stir everything together until the yoghurt is combined with the berries.

5. Add any other toppings you'd like, such as nuts, seeds, or granola.

6. Serve the yoghurt with berries and enjoy!

This yoghurt with berries recipe is a great way to start your day with a nutritious and delicious breakfast. Plus, it's low in calories and high in beneficial
Preparation time: 5 minutes

Baked sweet potato with grilled shrimp and steamed vegetables.

This recipe is a great option for those on a weight loss or dieting plan. It's full of healthy, low-calorie ingredients that are high in fibre and protein.

Ingredients:
- 2 sweet potatoes
- 2 tablespoons olive oil
- 1/2 teaspoon garlic powder
- Salt and pepper
- 1/2 pound raw shrimp, peeled and deveined
- 2 tablespoons fresh lemon juice
- 1/4 teaspoon paprika
- 2 cups of your favourite vegetables (broccoli, carrots, green beans, etc.)

Instructions:
1. Preheat the oven to 400 degrees F.
2. Pierce the sweet potatoes with a fork and place them on a baking sheet. Bake for 40 minutes or until they are tender when pierced with a fork.
3. In a large skillet over medium-high heat, warm the olive oil. Garlic powder, salt, and pepper are then added, along with the shrimp.
4. Add the lemon juice and paprika to the skillet and stir to combine.

5. Place the vegetables in a steamer basket over a pot of boiling water. Steam for 5-7 minutes or until the vegetables are tender.
6. Cut the sweet potatoes in half and top with the shrimp and steamed vegetables. Serve immediately.

Enjoy!
Preparation time: 20 minutes

Day 19

Breakfast

Smoothie bowl with banana, almond milk, and chia seeds.

Making a smoothie bowl with banana, almond milk, and chia seeds is a great way to add a healthy and nutritious breakfast to your weight loss and dieting routine.

Start by gathering all of your ingredients. You will need one banana, one cup of almond milk, and one tablespoon of chia seeds. Slice the banana into small pieces and place them into a blender. Add the almond milk and chia seeds and blend until it forms a thick and creamy mixture.

Once blended, pour the smoothie mixture into a bowl and top it with whatever additional fruits and nuts you would like. Popular choices include strawberries, blueberries, coconut, and almonds.

Finally, enjoy your smoothie bowl. The combination of banana, almond milk, and chia seeds provides a great source of protein and fibre, making it an ideal breakfast for those looking to lose weight and stay on track with their diet. Plus, it's delicious! Enjoy!
Preparation time: 10 minutes

Snack

A handful of nuts.

Making a handful of nuts is a great way to get the necessary nutrients and healthy fats while also maintaining a healthy weight and diet. Here is a simple guide to making a nutritious and filling handful of nuts:

1. Choose your nuts: Choose a variety of nuts to make your handful of nuts. Nuts like almonds, walnuts, pecans, cashews, and peanuts are all good choices.

2. Prepare the nuts: Make sure your nuts are clean and dry. If you're using raw nuts, you may want to lightly toast them in the oven or on the stovetop.

3. Measure out a handful: A good rule of thumb is to measure out a handful of nuts (about 1 ounce or 30 grams) for each person or serving.

4. Add flavour: If desired, you can add a sprinkle of salt or your favourite herbs or spices to your handful of nuts for a delicious flavour boost.

5. Serve: Place your handful of nuts in a bowl or on a plate and enjoy!

By following this simple guide, you can make a nutritious and satisfying handful of nuts that will help you maintain a healthy weight and diet. Enjoy!
Preparation time: 5 minutes

Lunch
Kale salad with grilled chicken, tomatoes, and balsamic vinaigrette.

Making a Kale Salad with Grilled Chicken, Tomatoes and Balsamic Vinaigrette is a great way to make a filling, nutritious meal that is perfect for weight loss and dieting. recipe to get you started:

Ingredients:

- 2 cups of fresh kale, washed and torn into small pieces
- 4 ounces of grilled chicken, cut into small cubes
- 1/2 cup of cherry tomatoes, halved
- 2 tablespoons of olive oil
- 2 tablespoons of balsamic vinegar
- Salt and pepper to taste

Instructions:

1. Heat a large portion of the skillet on low heat and add the olive oil
2. Add the chicken cubes to the skillet and cook until golden brown, about 5 minutes.
3. Add the kale to the skillet and cook for another 2-3 minutes until the kale is slightly wilted.
4. Remove the skillet from the heat and add the cherry tomatoes.
5. Balsamic vinegar and olive oil are put in a small bowl by mixing them.
6. Pour the balsamic vinaigrette over the salad and toss to combine.
7. Add salt and pepper to the food according to taste.
8. Serve the salad immediately and enjoy!
Preparation time: 15 minutes

Snack
Celery sticks with almond butter.

Making celery sticks with almond butter is a great way to enjoy a healthy snack while dieting or trying to lose weight. This snack is a great source of protein, healthy fats, and fibre, making it a nutritious and filling snack. Here's how to make it:

1. Start by washing and preparing your celery. Slice the celery into sticks and set aside.

2. Next, grab a bowl and add the almond butter. You can either buy or prepare your almond butter.

3. Using a spoon or spatula, mix the almond butter until it is smooth and creamy.

4. Take the celery sticks and spread the almond butter on each one. You can use a knife or spoon to make sure the almond butter is evenly distributed.

5. Once the celery sticks are topped with almond butter, you can enjoy them as is. You can also top them with other healthy toppings such as raisins, nuts, or seeds for extra flavour and nutrition.

This is a great snack for those looking to lose weight or eat healthily. The celery and almond butter provide a powerful combination of protein, healthy fats, and fibre.

Enjoy your celery sticks with almond butter for a nutritious and delicious snack

Preparation time: 5 minutes

Dinner
Baked salmon with sweet potato and steamed broccoli.

Ingredients

-4 salmon fillets

-1 sweet potato, peeled and diced

-1 head of broccoli, cut into florets

-2 tablespoons olive oil

-1 teaspoon garlic powder

-1 teaspoon paprika

-1/2 teaspoon salt

-1/4 teaspoon pepper

Directions

1. Preheat the oven to 400 degrees F.

2. Place the diced sweet potato on a baking sheet and drizzle with 1 tablespoon of olive oil. Add garlic powder and mix thoroughly. Bake for 20 minutes after placing in the oven.

3. While the sweet potato is baking, place the salmon fillets on a baking sheet and drizzle with 1 tablespoon of olive oil. Salt, pepper, and paprika should be added before tossing to coat.

4. Once the sweet potatoes have been baking for 20 minutes, add the salmon fillets to the baking sheet. Bake for 18 minutes after placing in the oven.

5. Place the broccoli florets in a steamer basket and steam for 8 minutes.

6. Once the salmon and sweet potatoes have finished baking, serve with the steamed broccoli and enjoy!
Preparation time: 20 minutes

Day 20

Overnight oats with banana and almond butter.
Making overnight oats with banana and almond butter is an excellent way to start your day off with a nutritious breakfast. Not only is it delicious, but it also helps promote weight loss and healthy eating.

To make overnight oats with banana and almond butter, you will need:

- ½ cup oatmeal
- ½ cup almond milk
- 1 banana
- 2 tablespoons almond butter
- 2 tablespoons chia seeds
- 1 teaspoon honey or maple syrup
- Pinch of cinnamon

Begin by adding the oatmeal to a bowl or jar. Add the almond milk and stir well to blend. Slice the banana and add it to the oatmeal.

Add the almond butter, chia seeds, honey or maple syrup, and a pinch of cinnamon. All the ingredients should be thoroughly mixed.

Cover the bowl or jar and place it in the refrigerator overnight. The next morning, your overnight oats with banana and almond butter will be ready to enjoy.

Overnight oats are a great way to start the day off with a nutritious meal that is low in calories, but high in fibre, protein, and healthy fats. The high-fibre content of the oats helps to promote weight loss and the almond butter and banana provide healthy fats and vitamins. Enjoy your overnight oats with banana and almond butter and start your day off right!
Preparation time: 10 minutes

Snack

Apple slices with a tablespoon of peanut butter.

To make apple slices with a tablespoon of peanut butter, first, wash and dry an apple. Cut off the stem and discard. Cut the apple into thin slices, about 1/4 inch thick. Place the slices in a row on a plate or board.

Take a tablespoon of creamy peanut butter and spread it over each apple slice. use crunchy peanut butter if you like. Sprinkle it with a pinch of sea salt for added flavour.

Enjoy your healthy snack. Apple slices with peanut butter are a great way to get your daily dose of protein, fibre, and vitamins. This snack is also perfect for weight loss and dieting. The natural sugars in the apple and the healthy fats in the peanut butter will help keep you feeling full longer, while the fibre and protein will help keep you energised throughout the day.

Preparation time: 5 minutes

Lunch

Turkey wrap with tomatoes, lettuce, and hummus.

To make a delicious and healthy Turkey Wrap with Tomatoes, Lettuce, and Hummus, follow these simple steps:

1. Start by gathering the ingredients: 2-3 slices of cooked turkey, 2-3 slices of tomato, a handful of lettuce, 2 tablespoons of hummus, and a wrap or tortilla of your choice.

2. Place the wrap on a flat surface, and spread the hummus evenly over the wrap.

3. Place the turkey slices in the centre of the wrap, followed by the tomato and lettuce.

4. Fold the wrap over the ingredients, tucking in the edges.

5. Heat a skillet over medium heat and add the wrap, cooking for 1-2 minutes on each side until lightly browned and crispy.

6. Slice the wrap in half and serve. Enjoy!
Preparation time: 10 minutes

Snack
Whole wheat crackers with cottage cheese.

Whole wheat crackers with cottage cheese are a great snack for weight loss and dieting. You can make them in a few simple steps.

1. Preheat your oven to 350 degrees

2. In a medium bowl, mix 1 cup of whole wheat flour, 1/2 cup of grated Parmesan cheese, 1/4 teaspoon of baking powder, and 1/4 teaspoon of garlic powder.

3. Add 1/4 cup of cold butter and mix until it is evenly distributed.

4. In a separate bowl, mix 1/2 cup of cottage cheese, 1/4 cup of olive oil, and 1/4 cup of water.

5. Now Add the wet ingredients to the dry ingredients and mix until everything is well mixed.

6. Roll the dough out on a lightly floured surface to about 1/4 inch thick.

7. Cut the dough into 2-inch squares and place them on a baking sheet lined with parchment paper.

8. Bake for 15-20 minutes, or until the crackers are golden brown.

9. Allow the crackers to cool before serving.

These whole wheat crackers with cottage cheese are a great snack for weight loss and dieting. They are high in protein, low in fat, and full of flavour. Enjoy!
Preparation time: 5 minutes

Dinner
Baked cod with steamed cauliflower and lemon.
Ingredients:

- 1 lb. cod fillet
- 1 head of cauliflower
- 2 tablespoons of olive oil
- 1 lemon
- Salt and pepper, to taste

Instructions:

1. Preheat your oven to 375°F.

2. Rinse and pat the cod fillet dry with a paper towel. Place the fillet on a baking sheet and season with salt and pepper. Squeeze half the juice of a lemon over the fish.

3. Cut the cauliflower into florets and place them in a large bowl. Salt and pepper to taste, then toss with the olive oil.

4. Place the cauliflower florets on a separate baking sheet and spread them out in an even layer.

5. Place both the cod and cauliflower in the oven and bake for 15-20 minutes or until the cod is cooked through and the cauliflower is tender.

6. Serve the cod with the steamed cauliflower and the remaining lemon slices. Enjoy
Preparation time: 15 minutes

Day 21

Breakfast
Scrambled egg whites with spinach and mushrooms.

Ingredients:
-1/2 cup egg whites
-1/4 cup mushrooms, sliced
-1/4 cup spinach, chopped
-1/4 teaspoon garlic powder
-Salt and pepper, to taste

Instructions:
1. Heat a non-stick skillet over medium-high heat.

2. Once heated, add the mushrooms and spinach and sauté for about 3 minutes until the mushrooms and spinach are softened.

3. Add the egg whites and garlic powder and cook for an additional 2-3 minutes, stirring occasionally.

4. Season with salt and pepper, to taste.

5. Serve and enjoy!
Preparation time: 10 minutes

Snack

A handful of nuts.

A handful of nuts is a great snack for weight loss and dieting. They are low in calories, high in protein, and provide a good source of healthy fats. Here are some tips on how to make a healthy and tasty handful of nuts:

1. Start by selecting your favourite nuts. Choose from almonds, walnuts, hazelnuts, cashews, and pistachios. You can also add some dried fruit to the mix such as cranberries, raisins, or dried apricots.

2. Roast the nuts in a preheated oven at 350°F for about 10 minutes. This will bring out the flavour and make them crunchier.

3. Place the roasted nuts in a bowl and mix in a tablespoon of olive oil, one teaspoon of sugar, and a pinch of salt.

4. Divide the nuts into individual servings and store them in an airtight container for up to one week.

5. Enjoy your handful of nuts as a snack throughout the day or as part of a meal.

These tips will help you make a healthy and tasty handful of nuts for weight loss and dieting. Enjoy!
 Preparation time: 5 minutes

Lunch
Quinoa bowl with grilled chicken, tomatoes, and balsamic vinaigrette.

Making a quinoa bowl with grilled chicken, tomatoes, and balsamic vinaigrette is an easy and delicious way to eat healthily while still getting all of the nutrients you need. This bowl is ideal for weight loss and dieting, as the combination of quinoa and grilled chicken provides a great source of protein while the tomatoes and balsamic vinaigrette add flavour and texture. Here is how to make it:

1. Begin by cooking the quinoa according to the package instructions.

2. While the quinoa is cooking, prepare the chicken by sprinkling it with salt and pepper and grilling it on both sides until it is cooked through.

3. Slice the tomatoes into thin slices and set aside.

4. In a small bowl, whisk together a tablespoon of olive oil, two tablespoons of balsamic vinegar, and a pinch of salt and pepper.

5. Once the quinoa is cooked, assemble the bowl by adding the quinoa to the bottom, followed by the grilled chicken, tomatoes, and balsamic vinaigrette.

6. Enjoy your quinoa bowl with grilled chicken, tomatoes, and balsamic vinaigrette! It's a nutritious and delicious meal that's perfect for weight loss and dieting.
Preparation time: 15 minutes

Snack
Celery sticks with almond butter.

Making celery sticks with almond butter is a great way to snack while dieting and trying to lose weight. Here is a simple recipe to make this tasty snack:

Ingredients:

-Celery sticks
-Almond butter

Instructions:

1. Cut the celery into 3-4 inch sticks.

2. Spread a thin layer of almond butter on each celery stick.

3. Place the celery sticks on a plate or in a container and enjoy!

Almond butter is a great choice for those on a diet because it is high in protein and low in sugar. The combination of celery and almond butter makes for a nutritious and satisfying snack. Enjoy!
Preparation time: 5 minutes

Baked sweet potato with grilled shrimp and sautéed vegetables.

Ingredients:

• 1 pound of peeled and deveined shrimp,
2 big sweet potatoes, cut into cubes, and
1 red bell pepper, cored and diced.
• 1 red onion, cut into wedges
• 1 zucchini, sliced
• 1 yellow squash, sliced
• 2 cloves garlic, minced
• 2 tablespoons olive oil
• 1 teaspoon sea salt
• 1 teaspoon black pepper
• 1 teaspoon dried oregano
• 1 teaspoon dried basil
• 2 tablespoons fresh parsley, chopped

Instructions:

1. Preheat your oven to 375 degrees

2. Place the cubed sweet potatoes onto a baking sheet and drizzle with 1 tablespoon of olive oil. Bake for 20 minutes or till well cooked

3. Meanwhile, heat the remaining 1 tablespoon of olive oil in a large skillet over medium heat. Add the shrimp, bell pepper, onion, zucchini, yellow squash, and garlic and sauté for 5 minutes.

4. Season the shrimp and vegetables with sea salt, black pepper, oregano, and basil.

5. Add the cooked sweet potatoes to the skillet and stir to combine.

6. Continue to sauté for 5 minutes or until the shrimp is cooked through.

7. Serve the baked sweet potato with grilled shrimp and sautéed vegetables garnished with fresh parsley. Enjoy!
Preparation time: 20 minutes

Day 22

Breakfast
Oatmeal with fresh fruit and nuts.

Making oatmeal with fresh fruit and nuts is a great way to get a healthy, nutritious breakfast that is perfect for weight loss and dieting. Here are the steps to making oatmeal with fresh fruit and nuts:

1. Start by measuring out one cup of dry oats into a medium-sized bowl.

2. Add two cups of water to the oats, and bring to a boil. Reduce the heat and simmer for 5-7 minutes.

3. Once the oats are cooked, add 1/4 cup of chopped nuts of your choice, such as almonds, walnuts, or pecans.

4. Add 1/2 cup of your favourite fresh fruit, such as berries, bananas, apples, or pears.

5. If desired, add a tablespoon of honey or maple syrup for extra sweetness.

6. Stir the ingredients together and let cool for a few minutes before serving.

Enjoy your oatmeal with fresh fruit and nuts for a healthy breakfast that is perfect for weight loss and dieting.

Happy eating!
 Preparation time: 10 minutes

Snack
Apple slices with peanut butter.

To make apple slices with peanut butter for weight loss and dieting, you will need the following ingredients:

-One apple
-One tablespoon of natural peanut butter

Instructions:

1. Start by washing the apple and cutting it into slices.

2. Spread the natural peanut butter on each apple slice.

3. Enjoy your delicious and healthy snack!

This snack is perfect for weight loss and dieting since it is low in calories and packed with nutritional benefits. The apples provide a great source of fibre, while the peanut butter is a healthy source of protein and healthy fats. Enjoy your apple slices with peanut butter as a snack or even as a quick breakfast.
Preparation time: 5 minutes

Lunch

Grilled chicken with quinoa and roasted vegetables.
Ingredients:

-2 boneless, skinless chicken breasts
-1 cup of cooked quinoa
-1 zucchini, cut into thin slices
-1 red bell pepper, cut into thin slices
-1 yellow bell pepper, cut into thin slices
-2 tablespoons olive oil
-1 teaspoon garlic powder
-1 teaspoon paprika
-Salt and pepper to taste

Instructions:

1. Preheat your outdoor grill or indoor grill pan to medium-high heat.

2. Place the chicken breasts on the grill and cook for 4-5 minutes per side, or until cooked through.

3. Meanwhile, toss the zucchini and bell peppers with olive oil, garlic powder, paprika, salt, and pepper in a large bowl.

4. Place the vegetables on the grill and cook for 4-5 minutes, or until tender and lightly charred.

5. To assemble the dish, divide the quinoa between two plates and top it with the grilled chicken and roasted vegetables. Enjoy!

Preparation time: 15 minutes

Snack
Yoghurt with berries.

Preparation time: 5 minutes

Dinner: Baked salmon with quinoa and roasted Brussels sprouts.
Ingredients:

-1/2 pound of salmon
-1/4 cup of quinoa
-1/2 pound of Brussels sprouts
-2 tablespoons of olive oil
-1 teaspoon of garlic powder
-1/2 teaspoon of dried oregano
-1/2 teaspoon of dried thyme
-1/4 teaspoon of salt
-1/4 teaspoon of pepper

Instructions:

1. Preheat your oven to 400 degrees F.

2. Arrange the salmon on a baking sheet and season with garlic powder, oregano, thyme, salt, and pepper.

3. Cook in the preheated oven for 10-12 minutes (or until the salmon is cooked through).

4. Meanwhile, bring 1/2 cup of water to a boil in a medium saucepan. Add the quinoa, reduce the heat to low, cover, and simmer for 10-15 minutes.

5. Trim the Brussels sprouts and cut them in half. Toss them with olive oil and spread them on a baking sheet.

6. Place the Brussels sprouts in the oven and roast for 15-20 minutes.

7. When the salmon and Brussels sprouts are done, serve them with cooked quinoa.

Enjoy your delicious baked salmon with quinoa and roasted Brussels sprouts!
Preparation time: 20 minutes

Day 23

Breakfast
Avocado toast with poached eggs.

Avocado toast with poached eggs is a delicious and nutritious meal that can be part of a healthy weight loss and dieting plan. To make it, you will need:

- 2 slices of whole-grain toast
- 1 ripe avocado
- 2 eggs
- Salt and pepper to taste

Instructions:

1. Start by toasting the two slices of toast.

2. Meanwhile, poach the eggs in a pot of boiling water. Once cooked, remove them with a slotted spoon and set aside.

3. Cut the avocado in half, remove the pit, and scoop out the flesh. Mash the avocado in a bowl and season with salt and pepper.

4. Spread the mashed avocado on the toast and top it with the poached eggs.

5. Serve the avocado toast with poached eggs and enjoy!

This delicious and healthy meal is a great way to get in some of the important nutrients that your body needs while still staying on track with your weight loss and dieting goals. Enjoy!
 Preparation time: 10 minutes

Snack
A handful of nuts.

A handful of nuts is a great snack for weight loss and dieting. They are low in calories, high in protein, and provide a good source of healthy fats. Here are some tips on how to make a healthy and tasty handful of nuts:

1. Start by selecting your favourite nuts. Choose from almonds, walnuts, hazelnuts, cashews, and pistachios. You can also add some dried fruit to the mix such as cranberries, raisins, or dried apricots.

2. Roast the nuts in a preheated oven at 350°F for about 10 minutes. This will bring out the flavour and make them crunchier.

3. Place the roasted nuts in a bowl and mix in a tablespoon of olive oil, one teaspoon of sugar, and a pinch of salt.

4. Divide the nuts into individual servings and store them in an airtight container for up to one week.

5. Enjoy your handful of nuts as a snack throughout the day or as part of a meal.

These tips will help you make a healthy and tasty handful of nuts for weight loss and dieting. Enjoy! Preparation time: 5 minutes

Lunch

Lentil soup with a side of whole wheat toast.
Lentil soup with a side of whole wheat toast is an excellent choice for weight loss and dieting. This dish is high in protein and fibre, which can help keep you fuller for longer and promote weight loss. Here's how to make it:

Ingredients:

-1 cup dry lentils
-1 onion, diced
-3 cloves garlic, minced
-2 carrots, diced
-1 celery stalk, diced
-2 tablespoons olive oil
-4 cups vegetable broth
-1 teaspoon ground cumin

-1 teaspoon dried oregano
-Salt and pepper to taste
-Whole wheat toast slices

Instructions:

1. Heat the olive oil in a large pot over medium heat. Add the onion, garlic, carrots, and celery and cook until softened, about 5 minutes.

2. Add the lentils, vegetable broth, cumin, and oregano. Bring to a boil then reduce heat, cover and simmer for 25 minutes.

3. Remove the soup from the heat and season with salt and pepper. Ladle the soup into bowls.

4. Toast the slices of whole wheat bread and serve with the soup. Enjoy!
Preparation time: 15 minutes

Snack
Celery sticks with almond butter.

Celery sticks with almond butter make a great snack for weight loss and dieting. Here's how to make them:

1. Start by washing and cutting three to four celery stalks into thin sticks.

2. Spread a tablespoon of almond butter evenly among the celery sticks.

3. Sprinkle a pinch of sea salt or a sprinkle of cinnamon on top of the almond butter.

4. Enjoy your snack!

These celery sticks with almond butter are a great snack for weight loss and dieting because they are low in calories and fat, and high in fibre and protcin. Thc almond butter adds healthy fats and some sweetness, helping to satisfy cravings. The sea salt or cinnamon adds just enough flavour to make the snack enjoyable without adding a lot of calories. Enjoy!
Preparation time: 5 minutes

Dinner
Baked cod with roasted Brussels sprouts and lemon.

Ingredients:

• 4 (4-6 oz) cod fillets

• 2 tablespoons extra-virgin olive oil

• 2 tablespoons freshly squeezed lemon juice

• 1 teaspoon garlic powder

• 1 teaspoon dried oregano

• 1 teaspoon dried thyme

• 1/2 teaspoon sea salt

• 1/4 teaspoon freshly ground black pepper

• 1 pound Brussels sprouts, trimmed and halved

• 2 tablespoons freshly squeezed lemon juice

Instructions:

1. Preheat the oven to 400°F.

2. In a small bowl, combine the olive oil, lemon juice, garlic powder, oregano, thyme, salt, and pepper.

3. Place the cod fillets in a baking dish and brush them with the olive oil mixture.

4. Place the Brussels sprouts around the cod.

5. Drizzle the lemon juice over the Brussels sprouts.

6. Bake for 20 minutes, or until the cod is cooked through and the Brussels sprouts are tender.

7. Serve immediately. Enjoy!
 Preparation time: 20 minutes

Day 24

Breakfast
Smoothie bowl with banana, almond milk, and chia seeds.

Making a smoothie bowl with banana, almond milk, and chia seeds is a great way to create a healthy and nutritious meal that can support weight loss and dieting. Here's how to make it:

1. Start by gathering all of the necessary ingredients – a banana, almond milk, and chia seeds.

2. Peel the banana and cut it into small pieces. Place the pieces in a blender and add the almond milk.

3. Blend the ingredients until they are fully mixed and smooth.

4. Pour the blended mixture into a bowl, and then sprinkle the chia seeds over the top.

5. Add any other toppings you would like, such as fresh fruit, nuts, or granola.

6. Enjoy your smoothie bowl and reap the benefits of all the healthy ingredients!

By combining the banana, almond milk, and chia seeds, you have created a delicious and nutritious meal that is perfect for weight loss and dieting. Enjoy!
Preparation time: 10 minutes

Snack
Apple slices with peanut butter.

To make apple slices with a tablespoon of peanut butter, first, wash and dry an apple. Cut off the stem and discard. Cut the apple into thin slices, about 1/4 inch thick. Arrange the slices on a plate or tray.

Take a tablespoon of creamy peanut butter and spread it over each apple slice. You can also use crunchy peanut butter if you prefer. Sprinkle it with a pinch of sea salt for added flavour.

Enjoy your healthy snack. Apple slices with peanut butter are a great way to get your daily dose of protein, fibre, and vitamins. This snack is also perfect for weight loss and dieting. The natural sugars in the apple and the healthy fats in the peanut butter will help keep you feeling full
longer, while the fibre and protein will help keep you energised throughout the day.
Preparation time: 5 minutes

Greek salad with grilled chicken, feta cheese, and olives.

Greek Salad with Grilled Chicken, Feta Cheese, and Olives is a delicious and healthy dish that can be enjoyed as a meal or a snack. Here is a simple recipe for this flavorful dish:

Ingredients:

- 2 boneless, skinless chicken breasts
- 2 cups chopped Romaine lettuce
- 1/2 cup Feta cheese, crumbled
- 1/2 cup pitted Kalamata olives
- 1/2 cup diced red onion
- 1/2 cup diced cucumber
- 1/4 cup olive oil
- 1 tablespoon fresh oregano, chopped
- 2 tablespoons fresh lemon juice
- Salt and pepper to taste

Directions:

1. Preheat the grill to medium-high heat.

2. Season the chicken breasts with salt and pepper. Grill the chicken for 5-7 minutes per side, or until the chicken is cooked through. Remove from the grill and let rest for 5 minutes before slicing.

3. In a large bowl, combine the Romaine lettuce, Feta cheese, olives, red onion, and cucumber.

4. In a small bowl, whisk together the olive oil, oregano, and lemon juice. Pour over the salad mixture and toss to coat.

5. Add the sliced chicken and toss to combine.

6. Season with salt and pepper to taste. Serve and enjoy.
Preparation time: 15 minutes

Snack
Whole wheat crackers with cottage cheese.

Ingredients:

-1 cup whole wheat flour
-1/4 teaspoon baking powder
-1/4 teaspoon garlic powder
-1/4 teaspoon onion powder
-1/4 teaspoon salt
-2 tablespoons olive oil
-3/4 cup cottage cheese
-3 tablespoons water

Instructions:

1. Preheat the oven to 375 degrees Fahrenheit.

2. In a medium bowl, mix the wheat flour, baking powder, garlic powder, onion powder, and salt.

3. Add the olive oil, cottage cheese, and water to the dry ingredients and mix until everything is well combined.

4. Place the dough onto a lightly floured surface and roll it out to about 1/4 inch thick. Cut into desired shapes using a cookie cutter or sharp knife.

5. Place the crackers on a lightly greased baking sheet and bake for 10-15 minutes, or until golden brown.

6. Let the crackers cool before serving. Enjoy!
Preparation time: 5 minutes

Baked sweet potato with grilled shrimp and steamed vegetables.

Ingredients:

- 2 sweet potatoes (about 8 ounces each)

- 2 tablespoons olive oil

- 1/4 teaspoon garlic powder

- 1/4 teaspoon paprika

- Salt and pepper

- 1 pound shrimp (peeled, deveined, and tails removed)

- 2 tablespoons olive oil

- 2 tablespoons fresh lemon juice

- 2 tablespoons fresh chopped parsley

- 2 cups mixed vegetables (such as broccoli, carrots, and cauliflower)

Instructions:

1. Preheat the oven to 400°F.

2. Cut the sweet potatoes into 1-inch cubes and place them on a baking sheet. Drizzle with olive oil, garlic powder, paprika, and salt and pepper to taste. Toss to coat. Bake for 25-30 minutes, stirring occasionally until the sweet potatoes are tender.

3. Meanwhile, in a large bowl, combine the shrimp with olive oil, lemon juice, parsley, and salt and pepper to taste. Toss to coat.

4. Heat a large skillet over medium-high heat. Add the shrimp and cook for 2-3 minutes, stirring occasionally, until the shrimp are cooked through.

5. Place the vegetables in a steamer basket over a medium saucepan filled with 1 inch of boiling water. Cover and steam for 3-5 minutes, until the vegetables are tender.

6. Serve the sweet potatoes with grilled shrimp and steamed vegetables. Enjoy!
Preparation time: 20 minutes

Day 25

Breakfast

Overnight oats with banana and almond butter.

Overnight oats with banana and almond butter are a great choice for weight loss and dieting. It's easy to make, nutritious, and filling. Here's how to make it:

Ingredients:
- 1/2 cup of rolled oats
- 1/2 cup of almond milk
- 1/2 banana, sliced
- 1 teaspoon of almond butter
- 1 teaspoon of honey

Instructions:
1. In a bowl, mix the oats and almond milk.
2. Add the sliced banana, almond butter, and honey.
3. Mix until everything is well combined.
4. Cover the bowl and place it in the fridge overnight.
5. In the morning, your oats are ready to be eaten. Enjoy!

Overnight oats with banana and almond butter are a great nutritious breakfast that will help keep you feeling full and satisfied throughout the day. Enjoy!
Preparation time: 10 minutes

Snack

Celery sticks with hummus.

Making celery sticks with hummus for weight loss and dieting is a simple and healthy snack. Here is how to do it:

1. Start by washing the celery sticks thoroughly.

2. Chop the celery sticks into smaller pieces, about 3-4 inches long.

3. Place the chopped celery sticks into a bowl.

4. Prepare the hummus by mixing 1 can of chickpeas, 1 garlic clove, 1/4 cup tahini, 1/4 cup olive oil, 1/2 lemon juice, 1 teaspoon of sea salt, and a pinch of cumin. Blend all the ingredients in a blender or food processor until creamy and smooth.

5. Place the hummus into a bowl and stir in a few tablespoons of water to thin it out.

6. Dip each celery stick into the hummus, making sure to coat it evenly.

7. Serve the celery sticks with hummus as a healthy snack.

This is a great snack to keep you feeling full while helping with weight loss and dieting. Enjoy!
Preparation time: 5 minutes

Lunch
Kale salad with grilled chicken, tomatoes, and balsamic vinaigrette.

Ingredients:

- 4 cups of chopped kale
- 2 chicken breasts
- 2 tablespoons of olive oil
- 2 large tomatoes, diced
- 1/4 cup balsamic vinegar
- 2 tablespoons honey
- 1/4 teaspoon garlic powder
- Salt and pepper to taste

Instructions:

1. Preheat your grill to medium-high heat.

2. Drizzle the chicken breasts with olive oil and season with salt and pepper.

3. Grill the chicken for about 5 minutes per side, or until cooked through.

4. Remove the chicken from the grill and let it cool for a few minutes before slicing it into thin strips.

5. In a large bowl, combine the kale, tomatoes, and chicken strips.

6. In a small bowl, whisk together the balsamic vinegar, honey, garlic powder, salt, and pepper.

7. Pour the dressing over the salad and toss to coat.

8. Serve the salad immediately or chill it in the refrigerator for later. Enjoy!
Preparation time: 15 minutes

Snack
A handful of nuts.

A handful of nuts is a great snack for weight loss and dieting. They are low in calories, high in protein, and provide a good source of healthy fats. Here are some tips on how to make a healthy and tasty handful of nuts:

1. Start by selecting your favourite nuts. Choose from almonds, walnuts, hazelnuts, cashews, and pistachios. You can also add some dried fruit to the mix such as cranberries, raisins, or dried apricots.

2. Roast the nuts in a preheated oven at 350°F for about 10 minutes. This will bring out the flavour and make them crunchier.

3. Place the roasted nuts in a bowl and mix in a tablespoon of olive oil, one teaspoon of sugar, and a pinch of salt.

4. Divide the nuts into individual servings and store them in an airtight container for up to one week.

5. Enjoy your handful of nuts as a snack throughout the day or as part of a meal.

These tips will help you make a healthy and tasty handful of nuts for weight loss and dieting. Enjoy!
 Preparation time: 5 minutes

Baked salmon with sweet potato and steamed broccoli.

Ingredients:

- 4 (4-ounce) salmon fillets
- 1 large sweet potato, peeled and cut into cubes
- 1 head of broccoli, cut into florets
- 1 tablespoon olive oil
- 1 tablespoon lemon juice
- 1 teaspoon Dijon mustard
- 1 teaspoon dried oregano
- 1/2 teaspoon garlic powder
- Salt and pepper to taste

Instructions:

1. Preheat the oven to 400°F.

2. Place the sweet potato cubes on a baking sheet and drizzle with 1 tablespoon of olive oil. Toss to coat.

3. Place the salmon fillets on top of the sweet potatoes and season with salt and pepper.

4. In a small bowl, combine the lemon juice, Dijon mustard, oregano, garlic powder, and remaining olive oil.

5. Drizzle the mixture over the salmon and sweet potatoes.

6. Bake for 20 minutes or until the salmon is cooked through and the sweet potatoes are tender.

7. While the salmon and sweet potatoes are baking, place the broccoli florets in a steamer basket over boiling water.

8. Steam for 5-7 minutes, or until the broccoli is bright green and tender.

9. Serve the salmon and sweet potatoes with steamed broccoli. Enjoy!
Preparation time: 20 minutes

Day 26

Breakfast
Scrambled egg whites with spinach and mushrooms.

Baked salmon with sweet potato and steamed broccoli
Preparation time: 10 minutes

Snack: Apple slices with a tablespoon of peanut butter.
To make apple slices with a tablespoon of peanut butter, first, wash and dry an apple. Cut off the stem and discard. Cut the apple into thin slices, about 1/4 inch thick. Arrange the slices on a plate or tray.

Take a tablespoon of creamy peanut butter and spread it over each apple slice. You can also use crunchy peanut butter if you prefer. Sprinkle it with a pinch of sea salt for added flavour.

Enjoy your healthy snack. Apple slices with peanut butter are a great way to get your daily dose of protein, fibre, and vitamins. This snack is also perfect for weight loss and dieting. The natural sugars in the apple and the healthy fats in the peanut butter will help keep you feeling full longer, while the fibre and protein will help keep you energised throughout the day.
 Preparation time: 5 minutes

Lunch

Quinoa bowl with grilled chicken, tomatoes, and balsamic vinaigrette.

Making a Quinoa Bowl with Grilled Chicken, Tomatoes, and Balsamic Vinaigrette is a great way to get a nutritious and delicious meal that is perfect for weight loss and dieting. Here's how to make it:

Ingredients:

-1 cup of quinoa
-1 cup of cooked, diced chicken breast
-1 cup of diced tomatoes
-1/4 cup of balsamic vinaigrette

Instructions:

1. Begin by preparing the quinoa. Rinse the quinoa in a fine-mesh strainer, then cook according to the instructions on the package.

2. Heat a skillet over medium heat, then add the chicken. Cook until the chicken is golden brown and cooked through, about 8-10 minutes.

3. Add the tomatoes and cook for an additional 2-3 minutes, stirring occasionally.

4. Remove the skillet from the heat and add the cooked quinoa. Stir to combine.

5. Divide the quinoa mixture among four bowls.

6. Top each bowl with the diced chicken, tomatoes, and balsamic vinaigrette.

7. Serve and enjoy!

This Quinoa Bowl with Grilled Chicken, Tomatoes, and Balsamic Vinaigrette is the perfect meal for weight loss and dieting. It's packed with protein, fibre, and healthy fats, which will keep you feeling full and satisfied. Plus, it's super easy to make!
Preparation time: 15 minutes

Snack

Celery sticks with almond butter

Making celery sticks with almond butter is a great way to lose weight and stay healthy. Here's how to make them:

1. Start by washing and drying a few celery stalks.

2. Cut the celery into smaller sticks about 4-5 inches in length.

3. Place the celery sticks on a plate or in a bowl.

4. Scoop almond butter into a small bowl and microwave for 15-20 seconds until the almond butter is spreadable.

5. Spread the almond butter onto the celery sticks.

6. Sprinkle it with a pinch of sea salt and enjoy.

Celery sticks with almond butter are a great snack for weight loss and dieting as they are low in calories but packed with nutrition. They are also a great source of vitamins and minerals such as Vitamin A, Vitamin C, and potassium. Almond butter provides a source of healthy fats and protein, helping to keep you full and satisfied for a longer period. Enjoy your celery sticks with almond butter as a healthy snack or a light meal.
Preparation time: 5 minutes

Dinner
Baked cod with steamed cauliflower and lemon
Ingredients:

- 2 cod fillets
- 1/2 head of cauliflower
- 2 cloves of garlic, minced
- 2 tablespoons of olive oil
- juice of 1/2 lemon
- 1/2 teaspoon of salt
- 1/4 teaspoon of black pepper

Instructions:

1. Preheat the oven to 375°F.

2. Cut the cauliflower into small florets, and place in a steamer basket. Place the basket over a pot of boiling water, and steam for 8 minutes.

3. Meanwhile, place the cod fillets in a greased baking dish. Top with minced garlic, olive oil, lemon juice, salt, and pepper.

4. Bake in a preheated oven for 15 minutes.

5. Remove from the oven, top with steamed cauliflower florets, and serve.

Enjoy!

Preparation time: 15 minutes

Day 27

Breakfast
Oatmeal with fresh fruit and nuts.

Making oatmeal with fresh fruit and nuts is a great way to start your day off right while also helping to support weight loss and healthy dieting. Here's how to make it:

1. Begin by measuring out 1/2 cup of old-fashioned oats. Place them in a pot with 1 cup of milk or non-dairy milk and 1 cup of water.

2. Bring the mixture to a boil, then reduce the heat and simmer for about 5 minutes, stirring occasionally.

3. While the oatmeal is cooking, prepare your toppings. Slice up some fresh fruit of your choice, such as bananas, apples, or berries. Toast some nuts, such as walnuts, almonds, or pecans.

4. When the oatmeal is done, turn off the heat and transfer it to a bowl. Top with your prepared fruit and nuts, plus some honey or maple syrup if desired.

5. Enjoy your delicious and nourishing oatmeal!

By making oatmeal with fresh fruit and nuts, you can easily enjoy a balanced breakfast that is high in fibre and protein, and low in fat and calories. This is sure to help support your weight loss goals and make healthy dieting a breeze!

Preparation time: 10 minutes

Snack

Handful of nuts.

A handful of nuts is a great snack for weight loss and dieting. They are low in calories, high in protein, and provide a good source of healthy fats. Here are some tips on how to make a healthy and tasty handful of nuts:

1. Start by selecting your favourite nuts. Choose from almonds, walnuts, hazelnuts, cashews, and pistachios. You can also add some dried fruit to the mix such as cranberries, raisins, or dried apricots.

2. Roast the nuts in a preheated oven at 350°F for about 10 minutes. This will bring out the flavour and make them crunchier.

3. Place the roasted nuts in a bowl and mix in a tablespoon of olive oil, one teaspoon of sugar, and a pinch of salt.

4. Divide the nuts into individual servings and store them in an airtight container for up to one week.

5. Enjoy your handful of nuts as a snack throughout the day or as part of a meal.

These tips will help you make a healthy and tasty handful of nuts for weight loss and dieting. Enjoy!
Preparation time: 5 minutes

Lunch

Grilled chicken with brown rice and steamed broccoli.

Ingredients:

-2 boneless, skinless chicken breasts
-1 cup brown rice
-1/2 cup broccoli florets
-2 tablespoons olive oil
-Salt and pepper, to taste

Instructions:

1. Preheat your grill to medium-high heat.

2. Rinse the chicken breasts and pat dry with a paper towel. Rub the chicken breasts with olive oil, and season with salt and pepper, to taste.

3. Place the chicken breasts on the preheated grill, and cook for about 4-5 minutes per side, or until cooked through.

4. Meanwhile, cook the brown rice according to the package instructions.

5. Steam the broccoli florets for about 3-4 minutes, or until tender.

6. Serve the grilled chicken with brown rice and steamed broccoli. Enjoy!
Preparation time: 15 minutes

Yoghurt with berries.

Making yoghurt with berries is an easy and delicious way to lose weight and maintain a healthy diet. Berries are low in calories and packed with antioxidants and other essential vitamins and minerals, making them an ideal snack or addition to any meal. Here is the step-by-step process for making yoghourt with berries:

1. Start by gathering the ingredients: Greek yoghurt, your favourite berries (strawberries, blueberries, raspberries, blackberries, etc.), and a sweetener of your choice (honey, agave nectar, etc.).

2. Clean and cut the berries. Slice or mash them as needed.

3. Mix the Greek yoghurt and sweetener in a bowl.

4. Add the berries to the yoghurt mixture and stir.

5. Place the mixture in the refrigerator for at least an hour to allow the flavours to blend.

6. Serve the yoghurt with berries once it has chilled.

This yoghurt with berries is a great way to satisfy a sweet tooth while still maintaining a healthy and balanced diet. The antioxidants and nutrients found in the berries are sure to give you a health and energy

boost, while the yoghurt provides a low-calorie and protein-packed snack. Enjoy
 Preparation time: 5 minutes

Dinner
Baked salmon with quinoa and roasted Brussels sprouts.

Ingredients:

-4 salmon fillets
-1 cup quinoa
-1 pound Brussels sprouts, trimmed and halved
-3 tablespoons olive oil
-Salt and pepper, to taste
-1 tablespoon lemon juice
-2 cloves garlic, minced
-2 tablespoons chopped fresh parsley

Instructions:

1. Preheat the oven to 400°F.

2. Line a baking sheet with parchment paper. Place the salmon fillets on parchment paper.

3. In a medium bowl, combine quinoa, Brussels sprouts, olive oil, salt, pepper, lemon juice, garlic, and parsley.

4. Spread the quinoa-Brussels sprouts mixture onto the baking sheet around the salmon.

5. Bake for 20 minutes, or until the salmon is cooked through and the Brussels sprouts are golden brown.

6. Serve the salmon with the quinoa and roasted Brussels sprouts. Enjoy!
Preparation time: 20 minutes

Day 28

Breakfast
Avocado toast with poached eggs.

Making avocado toast with poached eggs is a great way to enjoy a delicious and healthy breakfast. Poached eggs provide a great source of protein and healthy fats, while the avocado adds a creamy texture and plenty of vitamins and minerals. To make this meal, you'll need to start by poaching the eggs. Fill a pot with 2-3 inches of water and bring it to a simmer. Crack the eggs into small dishes and carefully slide them into the water. Poach the eggs for 3-4 minutes, or until the whites are set and the yolks are still runny.

Once the eggs are cooked, remove them from the water and set aside. Toast a slice of whole-wheat toast until lightly browned. Spread some mashed avocado on the toast. Sprinkle a pinch of salt and pepper onto the toast. Place the poached eggs on top of the avocado toast and sprinkle with some more salt and pepper.

For an added boost of nutrition, you can top the toast with some fresh spinach, tomato slices, or microgreens. Or, even better, you can make the toast with an egg-white omelette instead of poached eggs. This will reduce the fat and calorie content, but still provide a great source of protein.

Finally, enjoy your delicious and nutritious avocado toast with poached eggs. This meal is perfect for weight loss and dieting, as it is low in calories, high in protein, and full of healthy fats and vitamins.
Preparation time: 10 minutes

Snack
Apple slices with peanut butter.

Making apple slices with peanut butter is an easy and delicious snack that can be enjoyed while dieting and trying to lose weight. Here is how to make it:

1. Gather the ingredients: one apple, one tablespoon of natural peanut butter, and a knife.

2. Slice the apple into thin wedges.

3. Spread the peanut butter onto each slice of apple.

4. Enjoy!

Making apple slices with peanut butter is a healthy snack option that is high in protein, fibre, and healthy fats. It is also a great way to satisfy a sweet craving without going overboard on calories or sugar. This snack is great for weight loss and dieting, as it will help keep you feeling full and satisfied for longer.
Preparation time: 5 minutes

Lentil soup with a side of whole wheat toast.

Making Lentil Soup with Whole Wheat Toast for Weight Loss and Dieting

Ingredients:

- 2 tablespoons olive oil
- 1 onion, chopped
- 2 cloves garlic, minced
- 2 carrots, diced
- 1 celery stalk, diced
- 1 teaspoon paprika
- 1 teaspoon ground cumin
- 1 teaspoon ground coriander
- 4 cups vegetable broth
- 2 cups dried green or brown lentils, rinsed
- 1 bay leaf
- 2 tablespoons lemon juice
- Salt and pepper to taste
- 2 slices of whole wheat toast

Instructions:

1. Heat the olive oil in a large pot over medium heat.

2. Add the onion, garlic, carrots, and celery. Cook, stirring occasionally until the vegetables are softened, about 5 minutes.

3. Add the paprika, cumin, and coriander, and cook, stirring, for 1 minute.

4. Add the broth, lentils, and bay leaf, and bring to a boil. Reduce the heat to low, cover, and simmer for 25 minutes.

5. Remove the bay leaf, and stir in the lemon juice. Season with salt and pepper to taste.

6. Toast the bread slices in a toaster or under the broiler until golden brown.

7. Serve the soup with the toast on the side. Enjoy!
Preparation time: 15 minutes

Snack
Celery sticks with almond butter.
Making celery sticks with almond butter is a great way to snack while dieting and trying to lose weight. Here Is a simple recipe to make this tasty snack:

Ingredients:

-Celery sticks
-Almond butter

Instructions:

1. Cut the celery into 3-4 inch sticks.

2. Spread a thin layer of almond butter on each celery stick.

3. Place the celery sticks on a plate or in a container and enjoy!

Almond butter is a great choice for those on a diet because it is high in protein and low in sugar. The combination of celery and almond butter makes for a nutritious and satisfying snack. Enjoy!
Preparation time: 5 minutes

Baked cod with roasted Brussels sprouts and lemon.

This healthy and delicious baked cod with roasted Brussels sprouts and lemon is a great meal for anyone looking to lose weight and maintain a healthy diet.

To start, preheat your oven to 400°F and coat a baking sheet with non-stick cooking spray.

Next, take four 4-oz cod fillets and place them on the baking sheet. Sprinkle the cod with salt and pepper, then drizzle a tablespoon of olive oil over the cod.

In a separate bowl, combine 1/2 pound of Brussels sprouts (halved) with 1 tablespoon of olive oil and a pinch of salt. Toss the Brussels sprouts together until the olive oil coats them. Place the Brussels sprouts on the baking sheet next to the cod.

Slice a lemon and place the slices around the cod and Brussels sprouts.

Bake the cod and Brussels sprouts for 25-30 minutes, until the cod is cooked through and the Brussels sprouts are slightly browned.

Once the cod and Brussels sprouts are finished cooking, serve them with a lemon wedge for added flavour and zest.

This delicious and nutritious meal is great for anyone looking to lose weight and maintain a healthy diet. Enjoy!
Preparation time: 20 minutes

Day 29

Smoothie bowl with banana, almond milk, and chia seeds.

Ingredients:
- 1 large banana
- 1 cup almond milk
- 2 tablespoons chia seeds

Instructions:
1. Peel and cut the banana into slices.
2. Place the banana slices in a blender and blend until smooth.
3. Add the almond milk to the blender and blend until combined.
4. Add the chia seeds to the blender and blend until combined.
5. Pour the smoothie into a bowl and top with your favourite fruits and nuts.
6. Enjoy your Smoothie bowl!
 Preparation time: 10 minutes

Snack
A handful of nuts.
A handful of nuts is a great snack for weight loss and dieting. They are low in calories, high in protein, and

provide a good source of healthy fats. Here are some tips on how to make a healthy and tasty handful of nuts:

1. Start by selecting your favourite nuts. Choose from almonds, walnuts, hazelnuts, cashews, and pistachios. You can also add some dried fruit to the mix such as cranberries, raisins, or dried apricots.

2. Roast the nuts in a preheated oven at 350°F for about 10 minutes. This will bring out the flavor and make them crunchier.

3. Place the roasted nuts in a bowl and mix in a tablespoon of olive oil, one teaspoon of sugar, and a pinch of salt.

4. Divide the nuts into individual servings and store them in an airtight container for up to one week.

5. Enjoy your handful of nuts as a snack throughout the day or as part of a meal.

These tips will help you make a healthy and tasty handful of nuts for weight loss and dieting. Enjoy!
 Preparation time: 5 minutes

Greek salad with grilled chicken, feta cheese, and olives.

Ingredients:

- 1 lb boneless, skinless chicken breasts
- 2 tablespoons olive oil
- Salt and freshly ground black pepper
- 2 cups romaine lettuce, chopped
- 1/2 cup thinly sliced red onion
- 1/2 cup crumbled feta cheese
- 1/2 cup pitted Kalamata olives
- 1/2 cup chopped cucumber
- 1/4 cup chopped fresh parsley
- 1/4 cup extra-virgin olive oil
- 2 tablespoons freshly squeezed lemon juice
- 1 teaspoon dried oregano

Instructions:

1. Preheat the grill to medium-high heat.

2. Rub the chicken breasts with olive oil and season with salt and pepper. Place the chicken on the preheated grill and cook for 5 to 7 minutes per side, or until the chicken is cooked through.

3. Meanwhile, in a large bowl, combine the romaine lettuce, red onion, feta cheese, olives, cucumber, and parsley.

4. In a small bowl, whisk together the extra-virgin olive oil, lemon juice, and oregano.

5. Once the chicken is cooked through, let it rest for 5 minutes before slicing.

6. Add the sliced chicken to the salad and toss it with the dressing.

7. Serve the Greek salad with grilled chicken immediately. Enjoy!

 Preparation time: 15 minutes

Snack
Apple slices with a tablespoon of peanut butter.

Making apple slices with a tablespoon of peanut butter is an easy and delicious way to have a healthy snack. To begin, wash and core an apple. Slice it into thin slices and arrange them on a plate.

Next, take a tablespoon of peanut butter and spoon it onto each apple slice. Make sure to spread it evenly. You can also use almond butter or other nut butter if you prefer.

Once the peanut butter is spread on the apple slices, it's time to enjoy! This snack is great for weight loss and dieting because it is low in calories, rich in fiber, and packed with healthy fats.

The combination of the sweet apple and the salty peanut butter is a delicious snack that will fill you up and satisfy your sweet tooth. Plus, it is a great way to get some extra protein into your diet. Enjoy!
Preparation time: 5 minutes

Baked sweet potato with grilled shrimp and sautéed vegetables.

Ingredients:

• 2 large sweet potatoes

• 1 lb shrimp, peeled and deveined
• 2 tablespoons olive oil
• 2 cloves garlic, minced
• 1 red bell pepper, sliced
• 1 small onion, sliced
• 1 zucchini, sliced
• 1 teaspoon paprika
• 2 tablespoons fresh parsley, chopped
• Salt and pepper to taste

Instructions:

1. Preheat the oven to 400°F (200°C).

2. Prick sweet potatoes several times with a fork and place them on a baking sheet. Bake for 40-50 minutes, or until tender.

3. Meanwhile, heat 1 tablespoon of olive oil in a large skillet over medium heat. Add garlic, bell pepper, onion, zucchini, and paprika. Sauté for 5-7 minutes, or until vegetables are tender.

4. Add shrimp to the skillet and cook for 3-4 minutes, or until shrimp is pink and cooked through.

5. When sweet potatoes are done, split them in half and top each half with equal amounts of the shrimp and vegetable mixture.

6. Drizzle with remaining olive oil and sprinkle with parsley.

7. Serve warm.

Enjoy your nutritious and delicious meal!
Preparation time: 20 minutes

Day 30

Breakfast

Overnight oats with banana and almond butter.

Overnight oats with banana and almond butter are a nutritious and delicious way to start your day. This healthy breakfast option is packed with fiber and protein, making it a great choice for weight loss and dieting. Here's how to make it:

1. In a bowl, combine ½ cup of old-fashioned rolled oats, ½ cup of almond milk, and a pinch of salt.

2. Mash one banana into the mixture and stir until it's fully incorporated.

3. Place the bowl in the refrigerator and let it sit overnight.

4. In the morning, take the bowl out of the fridge and add a tablespoon of almond butter.

5. Give the mixture a good stir and enjoy.

You can also top your oats with a sprinkle of cinnamon, a few chopped nuts, or a drizzle of honey if you'd like. Enjoy your overnight oats with banana and almond butter and stay on track with your weight loss and dieting goals!

Preparation time: 10 minutes

Snack
Celery sticks with hummus.

Making celery sticks with hummus is an easy and nutritious snack for weight loss and dieting. Here's how to make it:

1. Start by washing the celery sticks and cutting them into 4-5 inch pieces.

2. Place the celery sticks on a plate and set aside.

3. In a food processor or blender, combine 1 can of chickpeas, 2 tablespoons of tahini, 1 clove of garlic, 2 tablespoons of lemon juice, 1/4 teaspoon of cumin, 1/4 teaspoon of paprika, and 2 tablespoons of olive oil. Blend until the mixture is smooth.

4. Spoon the hummus into a bowl and serve it with the celery sticks.

Enjoy your delicious and healthy snack! Celery sticks with hummus are a great way to get your daily intake of fiber and protein, as well as help you stay fuller for longer. It's also a low-calorie option for those looking to lose weight or maintain a healthy diet.

Preparation time: 5 minutes

Lunch
Kale salad with grilled chicken, tomatoes, and balsamic vinaigrette.

Making a Kale Salad with Grilled Chicken, Tomatoes and Balsamic Vinaigrette is a great way to get in your protein and leafy greens while on a weight loss and dieting plan. Here's how to make it:

1. Start by prepping your ingredients. Rinse the kale and remove the stems. Chop the kale into small pieces. Slice the tomatoes into wedges. Grill the chicken breast until cooked through.

2. In a bowl, mix the kale, tomatoes, and chicken.

3. In a small bowl, mix the balsamic vinegar, olive oil, garlic, salt, and pepper to create the vinaigrette.

4. Drizzle the vinaigrette over the salad and toss until everything is evenly coated.

5. Serve the salad chilled or at room temperature. Enjoy! Preparation time: 15 minutes

Snack
A handful of nuts.

A handful of nuts is a great snack for weight loss and dieting. They are low in calories, high in protein, and provide a good source of healthy fats. Here are some tips on how to make a healthy and tasty handful of nuts:

1. Start by selecting your favorite nuts. Choose from almonds, walnuts, hazelnuts, cashews, and pistachios. You can also add some dried fruit to the mix such as cranberries, raisins, or dried apricots.

2. Roast the nuts in a preheated oven at 350°F for about 10 minutes. This will bring out the flavor and make them crunchier.

3. Place the roasted nuts in a bowl and mix in a tablespoon of olive oil, one teaspoon of sugar, and a pinch of salt.

4. Divide the nuts into individual servings and store them in an airtight container for up to one week.

5. Enjoy your handful of nuts as a snack throughout the day or as part of a meal.

These tips will help you make a healthy and tasty handful of nuts for weight loss and dieting. Enjoy!
 Preparation time: 5 minutes

Dinner
Baked salmon with quinoa and roasted Brussels sprouts.

Ingredients:

- 6 ounces of wild-caught salmon
- 1 cup of cooked quinoa
- 1/2 cup of roasted Brussels sprouts
- 1 tablespoon of olive oil
- 1 teaspoon of garlic powder
- 1/2 teaspoon of paprika
- Salt and pepper to taste

Instructions:

1. Preheat the oven to 425 degrees Fahrenheit.

2. Place the salmon on a baking sheet lined with parchment paper.

3. Drizzle the olive oil over the salmon.

4. Sprinkle the garlic powder, paprika, salt, and pepper over the salmon.

5. Roast the salmon in the preheated oven for 12-15 minutes or until the salmon is cooked through and flakes easily with a fork.

6. Meanwhile, heat a medium-sized pan over medium heat.

7. Add the cooked quinoa and roasted Brussels sprouts to the pan and cook until heated through.

8. Serve the salmon with cooked quinoa and roasted Brussels sprouts. Enjoy!
 Preparation time: 20 minutes

Chapter 5

Staying Motivated

Losing weight and dieting can be tough! You may start off feeling motivated, but it's easy to lose that motivation as the months go by. To stay motivated, it's important to focus on the long-term goal and set realistic, achievable goals. tips to help you stay motivated:

1. **Celebrate small successes:** Celebrating small successes along the way will help you stay motivated and remind you of how far you have come. For example, if you've lost a couple of pounds, reward yourself with a new item of clothing or a night out.

2. **Stay connected**: Connecting with other people on a similar journey can help keep you motivated. Join a support group or an online community to chat with people who understand your struggles and can help encourage you.

3. **Keep records:** Keeping records of your journey is key to staying motivated. Use a food diary or an app to help you monitor your calorie intake and exercise routine. Seeing how far you have come and how close

you are to your goal can keep you motivated and on track.

4. **Exercise:** Exercise doesn't have to be boring. Make it fun by trying out different activities or joining a class or gym. Listening to music while you work out can also help make it more enjoyable.

5. **Reward yourself:** Set rewards for yourself to keep yourself motivated. For example, when you reach a certain goal, treat yourself to a massage or a day out.

6. **Stay positive:** The most important thing is to stay positive. Don't focus on the negative and remember to give yourself credit for the small successes.

Losing weight and dieting can be a long and difficult journey, but with the right motivation and support, you can achieve your goal. Good luck!

Summary of Weight Loss Diet

A weight loss diet is a diet that is specifically designed to help people lose weight. It is typically divided into two main categories: low-calorie diets, which are designed to reduce overall caloric intake, and low-fat diets, which are designed to reduce the amount of fat in the diet. Depending on the diet, additional dietary changes may be made, such as reducing carbohydrates, increasing fiber, and reducing sugar intake.

The goal of a weight loss diet is to create a calorie deficit, which is when more calories are burned than consumed. To do this, a person should consume fewer calories than they expend each day. This can be achieved by reducing caloric intake from food and beverages, and increasing physical activity.

When starting a weight loss diet, it is important to focus on healthy eating habits that are sustainable in the long term. This includes eating a balanced diet that includes plenty of vegetables, fruits, whole grains, lean proteins, and healthy fats. In addition, it is important to stay hydrated, get enough sleep, and limit added sugars, saturated fats, and processed foods.

Following a weight loss diet can help people reach their weight loss goals, but it is important to remember that it can take time and dedication to see results. It is also important to speak to a healthcare professional before starting any diet or exercise program.

Conclusion

In conclusion, weight loss and dieting are complex and challenging topics that require an individual to employ a multifaceted approach. By taking into account each individual's unique situation and goals, they can develop an effective plan that is tailored to their needs. This plan should include eating a balanced diet that is rich in whole foods and limiting processed foods, exercising regularly, and getting adequate sleep. Additionally, individuals should seek out emotional and social support to help them stay motivated and maintain their commitment to long-term lifestyle changes. Weight loss and dieting are challenging topics, but with the right approach and commitment, individuals can make lasting changes that will lead to improved health and well-being.